DANCING MADNESS

Conceived and Edited by Abe Peck
Art Direction and Design by Suzy Rice

Rolling Stone Press

Anchor Books
Anchor Press/Doubleday
Garden City, New York
1976

Library of Congress Cataloging in Publication Data

Main entry under title:

Dancing madness.

"A Rolling Stone Press book."
1. Ballroom dancing—Addresses, essays, lectures.
2. Discotheques.   I. Peck, Abe.   II. Rice, Suzy.
GV1751.D2   793.3'3

The Anchor Book edition is the first publication of Dancing Madness
Anchor Books edition: 1976

ISBN: 0-385-11478-8
Library of Congress Catalog Card Number: 75-38163

Copyright © 1975, 1976 by Straight Arrow Publishers, Inc.

CONTENTS

INTRODUCTION

Get Dancin'!" "Boogie Down!" "Keep on Bumpin'!" "Shame, shame, shame . . . if you can't dance, too." Dancing madness is back. There's been Tango, Flapper and Marathon Madness; Lindy-Hopping, Jitterbugging, Twisting; the whirling dervish dancing of Woodstock.

This time around it's disco.

Dime-store sociology explains why the mainstream is, as the Kay Gees say, "hustlin' wit' every muscle." Black style is more accessible to whites than it was during the Smoldering Sixties. Gay-bar dance culture is "hot." Dancers don't take PCP or anti-get-up-and-go drugs. The Structured Seventies demand steps and touching instead of a formless expression of ecstasy. And dancing is cheap recession entertainment.

Disco has special assets. It's democratic; an obscure label with the apt name of Wing and a Prayer put four studio musicians together to "cover" a Broadway show tune and hit with "Ease on down the Road." Disco is anonymous; shadowy dancers follow the rhythms of invisible musicians through darkened dance halls. Disco is economical; club owners pay $50 a night for DJs instead of $500 a night for live performers, and dancers party for less than the price of a concert ticket.

Of course, disco can be charged with being boring, banal and, especially, predictable. Here's Michael Kunze, the German producer of Silver Convention and cowriter of the group's Number One single, "Fly, Robin, Fly," admitting as much:

"When I went to the discos, I realized that all you needed was a strong bass line, a snappy snare drum sound and some coloring on top. It's very important to have a dynamic part and a melodic part." It should be noted that all the cuts on Silver Convention's *Save Me* album sound pretty much alike, and that the musicians are so low profile that their record company could not identify them when asked for a photo caption. It should also be noted that Kunze has successfully answered his own key question: "What will make the people dance?"

Which brings us to Tom Vickers, who compiled the Disco Stars section of *Dancing Madness* and who taught Michael Kunze how to do the line dance called the L.A. Hustle when Kunze visited San Francisco. Tom turned 26 as we were finishing this book, and his birthday party featured a living room's worth of nonstop dancers. And the songs that turned us out the fastest were disco: the familiar bass line, the Philadelphia sound horns, the crisp drums. A friend of Tom's put "predictability" in its proper perspective. "Disco," he yelled over a high-decibel rendition of "Dancing Machine," "is dependable."

In *Dancing Madness*, Ed McCormack dives into Manhattan's trendy Le Jardin disco to experience what Truman Capote called "this terrible churning, the whole place churning like a buttermilk machine." Vince Aletti explores the behind-the-scenes mechanics and economics of the boom. Frank Robertson visits a DJ in his disco lair, Tom Vickers asks the performers and producers about thrills, fads and flaws. *Rolling Stone* Associate Editor David Felton consults a self-proclaimed "doctor of discogenics" on the hazards of high steppin'. But that's the background information; the real fun involves using the dance instructions and seeing how easy these dances are to learn.

Open, for example, to the spread for the L.A. Hustle, where disco dance instructor Karen Lustgarten explains how to move backward and forward and side to side without trampling your neighbor. Or read her opening instructions for the N.Y. Hustle or the Bump, and then fan the pages and watch Robert Grossman's disco dolls take you through the breaks and turns. Then, if you're ready for more, analyze the charts that will show you the Continental and Latin Hustles.

Disco is not the only dancing madness loose in the land. The Puerto Rican and Brazilian rhythms of salsa music have turned the Big Apple into the Big Mango. The strains of Jamaican reggae are heard on every college campus. The funky gymnastics of *Soul Train* are inspirational at parties like Tom Vickers'.

To capture these dances, we approached some sources for their steps. Trombonist Willie Colon showed how to flow along with salsa. Legendary Jamaican vocalist Toots Hibbert demonstrated the Chuckie and the Ride-a-Bike. *Soul Train* regular Damita Jo Freeman leaped through the Lock, broke down the Breakdown and high kicked through the Scooby Doo.

There's a last side to this dancing triangle. A week before Tom Vickers' birthday party, I went to another one 3000 miles away. Jack Peckolick, my father, was celebrating his 75th birthday at a Yonkers restaurant. In the main room, a bandstand's worth of Guy Lombardo-style gentlemen played a medley of big band hits. There was cheek-to-cheek Fox Trotting, Lindy rug-cutting, cherry-pink-and-apple-blossom-time Cha-Cha dancing.

I sat 'em out.

Back in San Francisco, I read Marshall Rosenthal's "It Seems We've Stood and Danced like This Before" retrospective, and learned how these First Steps came about. Then I consulted the Wedding/Prom/Bar Mitzvah Survival Guide compiled by professional ballroom dance instructor Teddy Lee. At the 76th birthday party, the ballroom will be more a treat than a trial.

If you want to sit this one out, you can enjoy this book as a "spool table book," which is a coffee table book for the casual set. Watch the Grossman figures go by. Look at the pretty pictures. Learn about Disco 'Round the World. Argue with our choices for the Keep on Dancin' All-Time Jukebox. Collect the set of Disco Star cards (sorry there's no chewing gum, but our publisher is Doubleday, not Double Bubble).

But if you don't dance through *Dancing Madness*, you'll miss a good time. So, in parting, let me offer you the wisdom of the Disco Kid. When Cindy McEhrlich, whose adventures in disco dance class earned her that nickname, was asked, "Doesn't it get boring?" her answer was simple, direct and true: "Watching is not the point. Watching is boring."

Abe Peck
December 1975

SECTION I

DANCING MADNESS

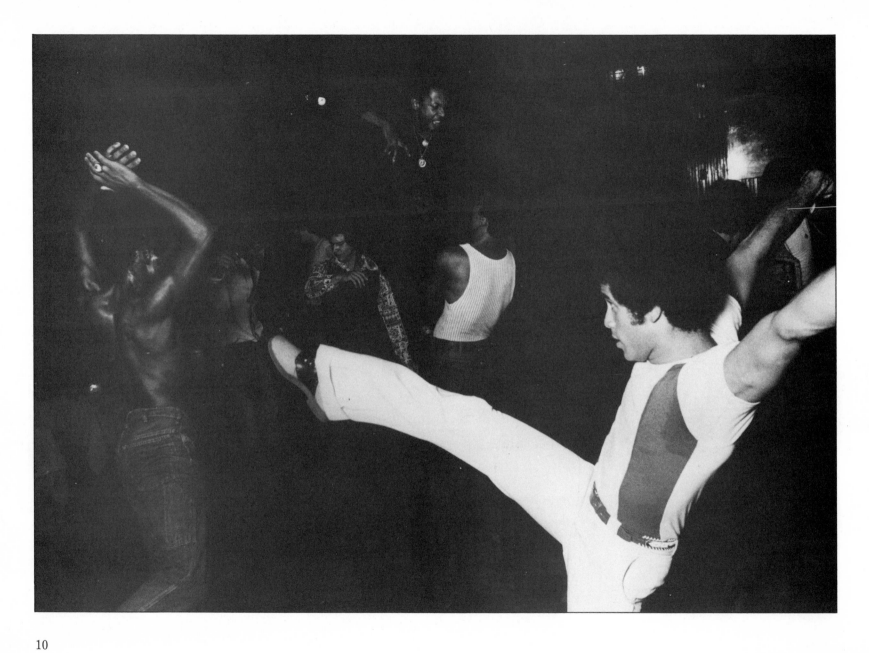

"NO SOBER PERSON DANCES"

In Which a Suburban Prole Decadent Visits a Hot Manhattan Disco and Learns that Cicero Was Right
by Ed McCormack

Never go to Le Jardin on the weekends," say the jaded, hipper-than-thou Wednesday night regulars—the boys who cut hair at Cinandre and the girls who readily confess to being "professional fag hags." After all, that's when all the novice prole decadents in platform heels and marshmallow clodhoppers come pouring in from the suburbs like some raging epidemic, and you need a tube of K-Y jelly to ooze into the penthouse-bound elevator of the gone-to-seed Diplomat Hotel on Manhattan's West 43rd Street. "Forget about the dance floor, honey," they warn, unless you're willing to risk the pumping, thumping, gang-banging glitter trash and hoi polloi who think that true art deco decadence can be purchased at the closest unisex boutique. "Believe me, baby," they advise, "your best bet is to try to talk your way into one of the private clubs"—because, they feel, even on these Wednesday nights the commuters from the outer boroughs have you surrounded, and no matter that Barry White is breathing in your ear like an obscene phone caller turned up to 110 decibels.

But if you chance the elevator's housing-project urine-odor ride upstairs and pay your $6 ($2 more if you're unhip enough to attend on weekends), you enter a totally other environment, the kind of place that, Truman Capote gushingly told a chin-in-hand Johnny Carson, has "these art deco couches all along the room, these palm fronds drooping down everywhere—and out on the dance floor this terrible churning, the whole place churning like a . . . buttermilk machine." At Le Jardin, the music commands a snaking daisy chain of dancers through pelvic puppet paces as the atmosphere grows heady with the adrenalin incense of Brut cologne and a thousand amyl nitrate poppers, each lending its queasy aphrodisiac rush to the whole

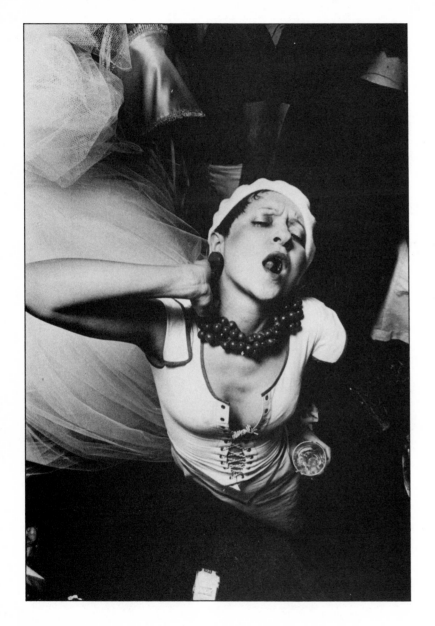

mind-boggling, switch-hitting group grope going on out there on the floor. After all, this is the place where the gamut of dress runs from Pierre Cardin suits to silver cosmic clothing, from Halston originals to backless halters, through all the shades, cycles and fetishes of chic, camp and queer, until it culminates in the truly bizarre ensemble of one muscular young madman who sports a leather aviator's cap, smoked Captain Midnight goggles and red plastic clothespins clamped onto his bare nipples, squeezing them out into two little ouch-drops of excruciating S&M ecstasy while he goes limpidly gazonkers out on the dance floor.

The crowd at Le Jardin is a mix of jaded Manhattan scene-makers like Hollywood DiRusso, a publicist in the New York office of famous Mod fashion figure Mary Quant, who checks out the disco action as soon as business takes her to a new city; mucho macho types like light-weight contender Chu Chu Malave, the Puerto Rican Mick Jagger of pugilism, who can frequently be spotted going through some Rudy Nureyev moves with his girlfriend, German model Uschi Odermier; boys who affect the smug upwardly mobile suave of Geraldo Rivera and girls who look like Carmen Miranda as drawn by *Interview* illustrator David Cryland and shake a spacey spice into the sometimes predictable syncopations of Soul Dancing; David Jo Hansen, former lead singer of the New York Dolls; Cyrinda Foxx, platinum-tressed sweater-girl starlet of the Seventies; Arthur Bell, who introduced gay activism to the New Journalism; and the members of a prole decadent generation weaned on cave-chested, Beardsleyesque Englishmen who shook their satin little buns like the swishiest

---

Hollywood DiRusso: "We all see ourselves as the Disco Queen— we're all out there to be noticed, to be . . . discovered."

of queens while bellowing as though the testicles of Muddy Waters had been grafted where his tonsils used to be, and who now find their way here, even on Wednesday evenings.

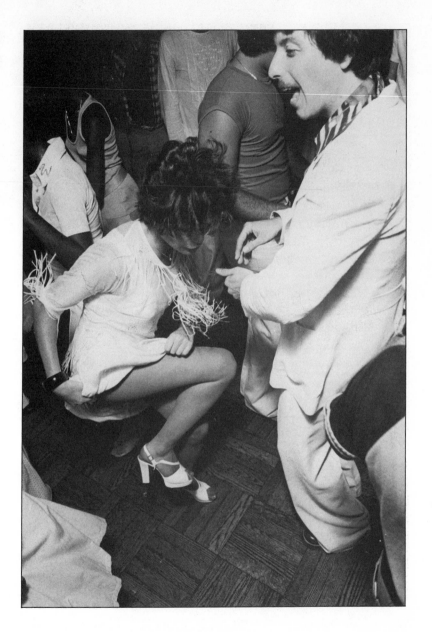

Take a kid like Tony Pagano, from Dongan Hills, Staten Island. They have more Civil Service people, minor Mafiosi and beat cops per square inch in Tony Pagano's home borough than in a 300-page Jimmy Breslin novel. These folks, mostly Irish and Italian drinking-class people, take a certain pride in having provided their offspring with modest, pastoral preserves that feature plaster saints on the mantle and pink flamingos on the lawn; you can imagine what Tony's poor parents must think when he puts on his Lou Reed T-shirt, his Mick Jagger pajama bottoms and his corkscrew wedgie sandals and lights out for 43rd Street.

"What my old man doesn't understand is that you don't have to be a fag to be into this scene," Tony says as he sips a tequila sunrise at the big, white leather bar behind which guys in basketball uniforms bound back and forth filling orders for drinks (the first test for the hetero male who wishes to be in tune with at least the basics of bisexual chic is to not feel threatened when addressed as "baby" rather than "sir"). "My old man doesn't understand that dancing is not a tight-assed, uptight sex role scene. It's just a way of communicating with people you might not have anything to say to if you sat down to talk. It doesn't mean you want to fuck a broad or a guy if you dance with them. You're just doing what comes natural."

But not to some. Le Jardin was "une discotheque pour monsieur" when it opened four or five years ago, and it stayed that way until Steve Ostrow, one of the more visionary gay entrepreneurs, came to terms with the specter of bisexual chic and set a precedent by opening his Continental Baths to women. Even today, this New Chicness remains as puzzling to older gays as it does to older straights. One vested, white-suited,

Carl Sandburg-haired Hollywood scriptwriter, who wrote for Joan Crawford and who goes back to the era when men in tuxedos danced tentative tangos in the furtive stag speakeasies of Hollywood Babylon, has retreated from the public befuddlement of the dance floor. Now, standing by the bar, he confesses his utter amazement: "Why, this is utterly shocking!" he says. "In my day, they would never have allowed a mixed couple in a gay dance establishment."

Then again, now is Now, and as Bobby DJ, a star in his own right, works the board with the intense concentration of a traffic controller to make Disco-Tex and the Sex-O-Lettes "get dancing" Hollywood, an indigenous scenemaker, a subterranean celebrity in the Warhol mold, takes to the dance floor.

"I make a decent salary, honey," Hollywood said later, "but at least three-quarters of it goes for rent and the rest I spend on discotheques dancing my cute little tush off."

Hollywood lives in a luxury high-rise in midtown Manhattan, but spends most of her nonworking hours in places like Twelve West and Le Jardin. "My philosophy is that you don't get discovered sitting at home. And let's face it: Everybody wants to be discovered for . . . something. I mean, every Eyetalian princess who goes dancing as much as I do—we all see ourselves as the Disco Queen—we're all out there to be noticed, to be . . . discovered! I'm such a severe case that I'm about to take a second job as a cigarette girl at Twelve West. Oh, it's going to be just fabulous. I wear a tiny little skirt and one of those campy cigarette-girl trays, you know, but it will be a small one so it won't be in the way when I dance!"

In her middle 20s, Hollywood caught the fever while still a teen. "I had already made up my mind to become a fag hag, but, as you can imagine, honey, Texas wasn't exactly what you would call a hotbed of flaming faggotry. I managed to sniff out the one or two gay bars in Dallas where you could go dance and . . . well, the very first time I just looked down at my feet and said, 'Honey, this is for you! This is it! This is even better than sex!'

"I mean, even though I'll go out on the dance floor and hitch my dress up over my head so you might—if you're lucky, boys —even see a flash of beaver, believe it or not I still go to church every Sunday. It's only a couple of blocks away from Le Jardin, and if I still went on weekends, I could dance out there and into early Mass."

Piety aside, Hollywood's concern with dancing feet has convinced her that the primary erogenous zone is the shoe.

"When a guy comes up to me and says, 'Do you wanna dance?,' the first thing I look at—even before the face—is the shoes. If I see a tacky pair of platforms or grotesque, chartreuse marshmallows, forget it, honey. But if I look down and see a nice pair of pumps, then I know that here is a guy with some awareness of elegance. Even penny loafers turn me on —I mean, those soft blue shoes you have on—ummm, I could rub my face all over those. . . ."

If such are the joys of being a Disco Queen, what possible drawbacks can there be?

"Well," Hollywood suggests, "one of the problems is that you have to master the art of looking bored. And that's pretty hard to do when you're really dancing and it's just building and building like an unending multiple orgasm. . . ."

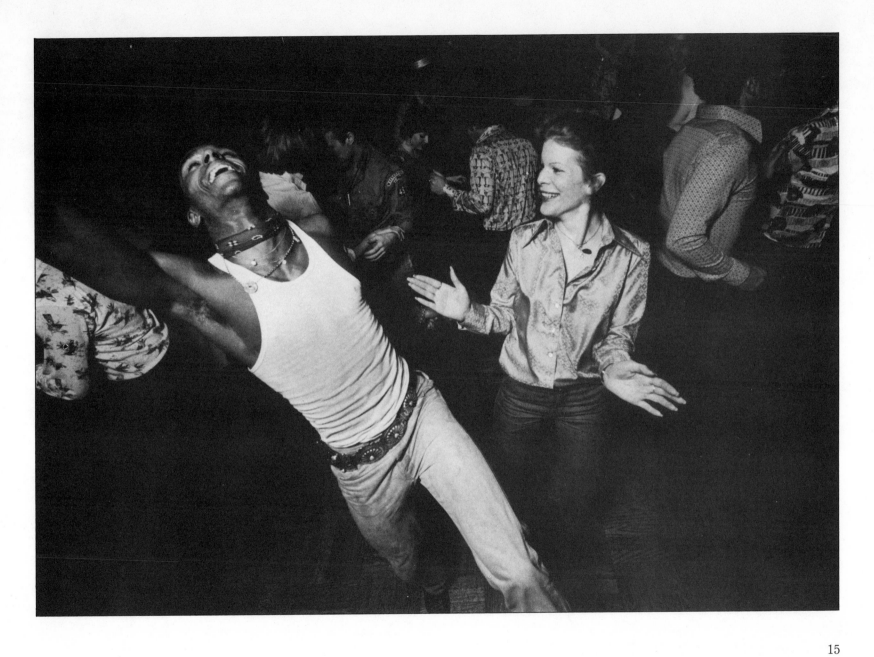

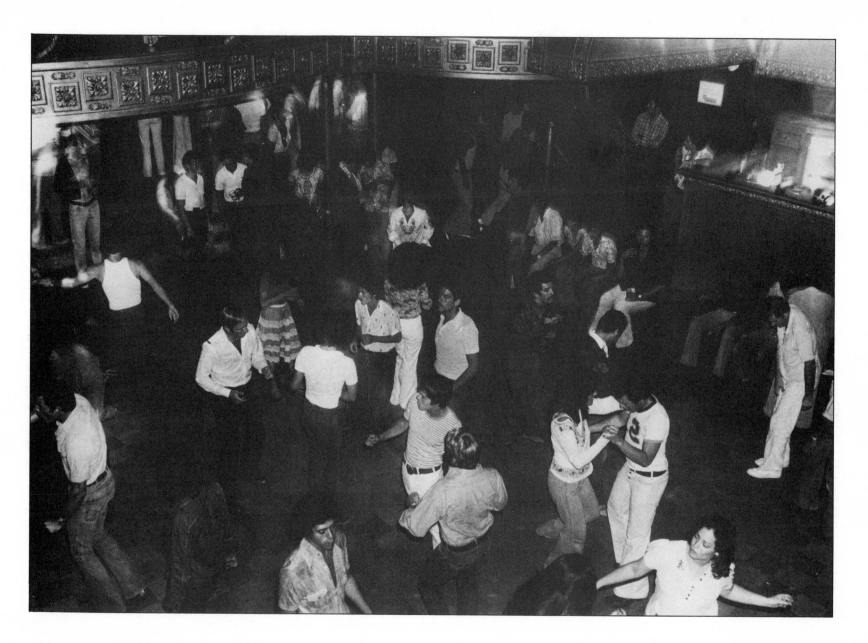

16

THE METHOD BEHIND THE MADNESS

Disco Madness Analyzed... The Disco Sound Revealed...
Some All-Time Disco Platters
by Vince Aletti

It's not easy to pin down the disco craze with figures. As one independent mixer of disco singles explained, "The numbers are growing so fast. Every day I get four or five invitations to grand openings of new clubs." But even the rough estimates of disco scene observers are revealing: 2000 discos from coast to coast, 200 to 300 in New York alone—the uncrowned capital of dancing madness, where an estimated 200,000 dancers make the weekly club pilgrimage. And when disco people like a record, it can become a hit—regardless of radio play. Take Consumer Rapport's "Ease on down the Road." Released on tiny Wing and a Prayer Records, it sold more than 100,000 copies in New York during its first two weeks—before it was picked up on the radio.

Discos and what has come to be known as disco music have turned out to be, if not the Next Big Thing everyone was anxiously scanning the music business horizon for, then the closest thing to it in years. Discotheques have opened up all over the country: in Baltimore and St. Louis and Fort Lauderdale and Phoenix, in old warehouses, steak restaurants, lofts, unused hotel ballrooms, failing singles bars—any place you could stick a battery of speakers, a ceilingful of flashing colored lights, a mirrored ball, two turntables, a mixer and a DJ. In a recession economy, discotheques are a bargain for both the club owner—who has few expenses after his initial setup investment and a nightly salary for the DJ (which averages $50, though some make nearly twice that much)—and the patron, who can dance all night for a fraction of the cost of a concert ticket (and with no worries about tuneup delays, cancellations, off nights, short sets, bad seats, unruly police, etc.). A good discotheque is the perfect, total-immersion environment for hearing music. The sound is intense, nonstop, loud enough to command total attention (sometimes loud enough to be literally

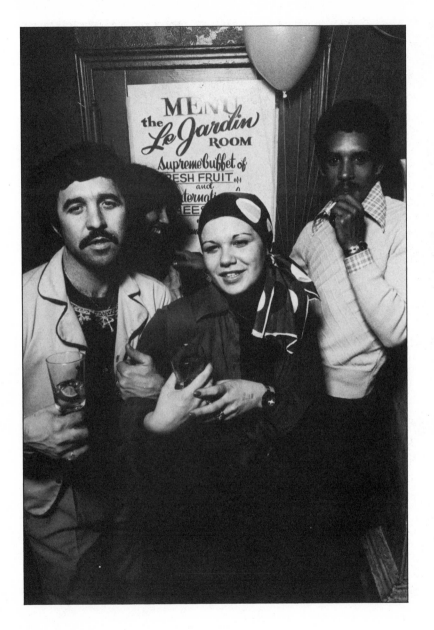

stunning) but relatively distortion-free. A talented DJ knows how to blend and place records in the flow-through course of an evening so that each one has maximum impact.

But the spread of disco music, especially since the middle of 1973, has outpaced even the growth of discotheques themselves. "Soul Makossa," by African singer Manu Dibango, was an early indication; Barry White's "Love's Theme," an even better one—it was discovered in discotheques six months before it hit the top of the national charts early in 1974. But it wasn't until later that year, when the Hues Corporation's "Rock the Boat" and George McCrae's "Rock Your Baby" were racing each other up the singles charts—and taking the Number One spot in quick succession—that the music business really began to take notice.

When companies realized that a fast-breaking disco record could jump from New York discos to key radio stations—well, there were no longer merely discotheques, there was the Discotheque Market. Suddenly everyone had a "disco" record, a "disco" album, a "disco" promotion man. There were "disco mixes," "disco versions," "disco series" with their own "disco" logos, special advance pressings marked "For Disco DJs Only." Following Barry White's lead, many singles were released with both vocal and instrumental sides or in a Part I/Part II format, with Part II being the "instrumental version" of Part I (meaning the vocal track was dropped) or, even better, the "long version."

Though the new disco music evolved from the hard dance records of the Sixties—primarily Motown and James Brown—the direction has been away from the basic, hard-edged brassy style and toward a sound that is more complex, polished and sweet. If one style dominates now, it's the Philadelphia sound, which is rich and elegant, highly sophisticated and tightly structured but full of punch. The Philadelphia producers are

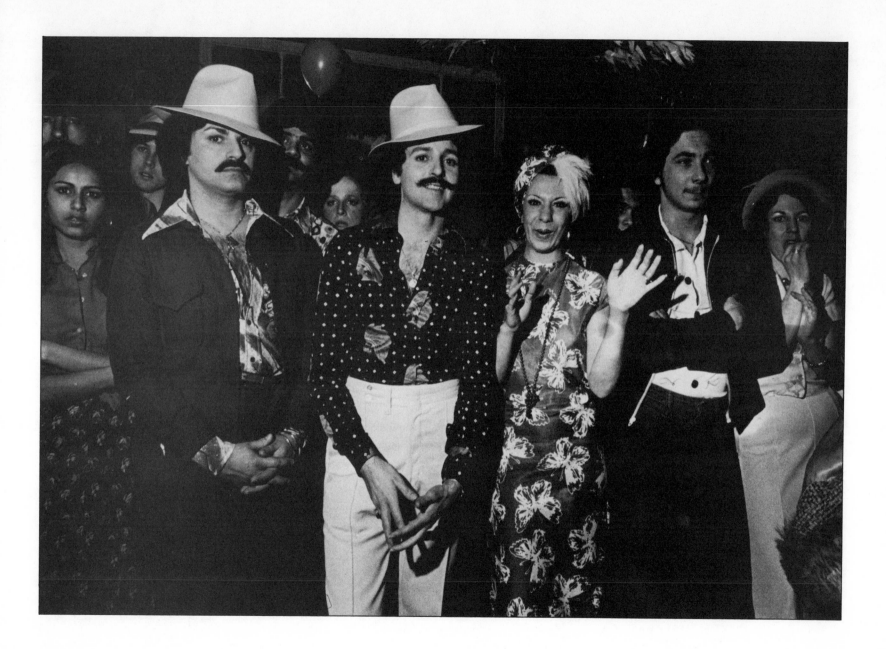

19

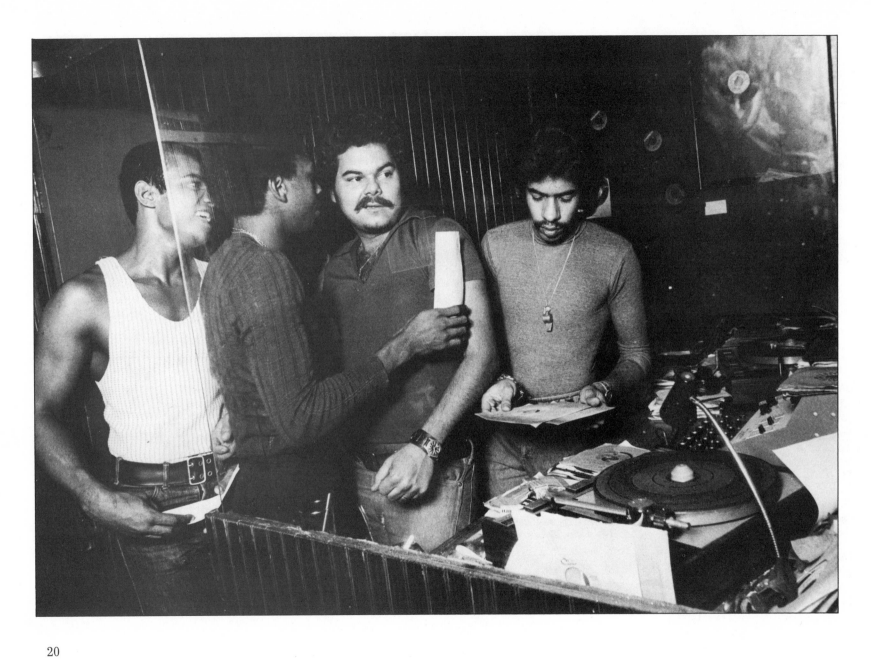

masters at using strings energetically, to boost as well as soften the arrangements, and they've perfected this glossy sound with Harold Melvin & the Blue Notes, the O'Jays, the Trammps, the Three Degrees and Blue Magic. Gamble & Huff and the other busy producers working out of Philly have also excelled in keeping their songs lyrically sharp and involving, while much other disco music has reduced lyrics to repeated words or simple verses. But disco music now includes so many different performers—from the Jackson 5 to Frankie Valli—and so many different styles, tied together only by a consistent danceable beat, that its definition has to be a broad one.

The discotheques' most obvious influence on music has been in the length of records. The best disco music is full of changes and breaks which allow for several shifts of mood or pace within one song and usually open up long instrumental passages. If the break works, it becomes the pivot and anticipated peak of the song—like the central one in Eddie Kendricks's "Girl You Need a Change of Mind," still one of the best dance records ever made or, more recently, the sudden burst of vocals in the middle of Crown Heights Affair's fine "Dreaming a Dream"—and the point of maximum excitement on the dance floor. It's hard to develop an effective build and break within a short record—it's just too abrupt and perfunctory and the mood on the dance floor is more leisurely, more indulgent. As long as the beat is tight and involving, and the texture of the changes is rich and diverting, a song can run six or eight or even ten minutes. So "disco version" or "disco mix" means, primarily, that the record is longer than the version released for radio play.

It may also mean that the cut has been specially mixed for a "hotter," brighter sound. Because discotheque DJs, much more than their radio station counterparts, are very concerned with the technical quality of the records they play, they reject some otherwise danceable singles because of the deadness of their mix or their loss of distinction at high volumes. This passion for quality sound has also had its influence on the record business: Several companies have put selected single cuts on 12-inch discs at 33⅓ for best reproduction at top volume.

Although all this attention has meant recognition at last for a number of performers who'd previously been trapped in the disco underground, it's also meant that much new "disco" music is merely a replay of several formulas that came before: the Barry White formula, the George McCrae formula, the Gloria Gaynor formula, etc. Much of the vitality of the sound has been carefully reduced to a few recognizable patterns that are shuffled and reshuffled into increasingly predictable disco ready-mades.

The disco-inspired revival of instrumentals has opened the door to a number of jazz artists who had never before enjoyed such wide exposure (like Grover Washington, Hubert Laws, Donald Byrd, Herbie Mann) but it's also let us in for albums like *Disco Party* by Percy Faith and Peter Nero's *Disco, Dance and Love Themes of the 70s*, both of which hang up a few superficial trappings of the disco sound without brightening the listless muzak underneath. Even Herbie Mann followed the most successful single of his career, a glossy cover of Barrabas's "Hijack" (at the time unreleased in this country), with an album called *Discotheque* (Atlantic SD 1670) that, while attractive enough, betrayed an almost total lack of comprehension of disco music, much less of a disco concept album.

Even if the disco scene eventually self-destructs on its own success, it remains diverse and open enough to revitalize and redirect itself. Disco DJs—the people who made all the musical connections in the first place, pulling together the different sounds that make up the total disco sound—are too adventurous to be pinned down to music biz definitions of disco. Already they've gotten heavily into European imports like Banzaii's "Chinese Kung-Fu" and Bimbo Jet's "El Bimbo." And there are so many young producers hooked into the disco sound that the ready-made formulas may fall by the side.

The following albums form a basic disco library—supplemental to the selected works of the O'Jays, the Temptations, Stevie Wonder, Earth, Wind & Fire, et al., but essential to anyone who wants to get to the heart of the music. Some of these records have already become disco classics; others may have passed from the current turntable repertoire. But all of them revive remarkably well given the right atmosphere.

Disco's Funky 15: A Basic LP Library

BARRABAS
Heart of the City

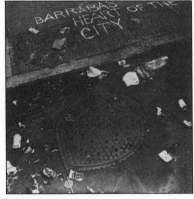

Acto SD36–118. The best album from a six-man Spanish group already responsible for a number of disco classics ("Wild Safari," "Woman," "Hijack"), *Heart of the City* is also a prime example of the European eclectic style at its most accessible. The vocals are rock style, rough, but the music ranges all over, taking Latin, jazz, Philly soul and L.A. rock elements and arranging them in all possible combinations. Particularly effective: "Family Size," "Checkmate," "Along the Shore" and a coolly refreshing instrumental called "Mellow Blow."

MFSB
Love Is the Message and Universal Love

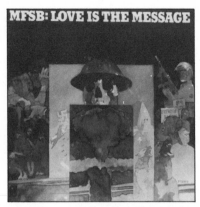

Philadelphia International KZ32707 and KZ33158. This is the Sigma Sound Studio house band, the Philadelphia musicians behind many of the groups on this list, the backbone of the Philadelphia sound. "TSOP," the former *Soul Train* theme, is the snappiest song on the first album, but the title track is deeper, even more of a pure disco classic. *Universal Love* may not cut quite as deep, but it's more consistent, more listenable and highlighted by "Sexy," "T.L.C." and "K-Jee." Like two boxes of rich chocolate.

BOHANNON
Keep on Dancin' and Insides Out

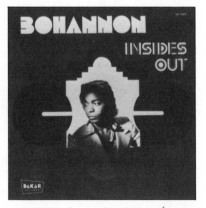

Dakar DK76910 and DK76916. The most distinctive and intriguing of the disco instrumentalists, Bohannon is a former Motown studio musician who was certainly never allowed to get this weird on Berry Gordy's time. The cuts are pushed to the limit (most of his are between five and seven minutes long), though he usually falls into an easy groove and holds to it relentlessly, adding a few sparse vocals which sound like cooled out tribal calls from the sophisticated urban jungle. Somehow it's all simultaneously boring and compelling. Start with the title cut, "South African Man," and "Truck Stop" on *Keep on Dancin'*, then sink into "Foot-Stompin' Music" and "Disco Stomp" on *Insides Out*.

B. T. EXPRESS
Do It ('Til You're Satisfied) and Non-Stop

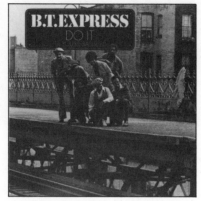

Scepter/Roadshow SPS5117 and RS–41001. The very best of the hard-edged, brassy New York City sound, from the first album's steamy, chugging instrumental "Express" (an instant classic) to "Peace Pipe" on the second, whose message combined peace and dope in a heady mix—the repeated chorus: "Put it in your peace pipe, smoke it all up." The disco hardcore love it.

ECSTASY, PASSION & PAIN

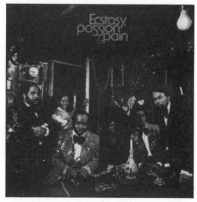

Roulette SR3013. A tough, screaming "girl group" sound from what is actually a two-woman, four-man band led by vocalist/guitarist/songwriter Barbara Roy — who sounds like a combination of Tina Turner and early Martha Reeves. Made in Philadelphia with the cream of MFSB, the album includes the group's three hottest singles—from the rising fever of "I Wouldn't Give You Up" to "Good Things Don't Last Forever" (a theme song for our

times) to the peak "Ask Me." Detroit 1964 meets Philadelphia 1974 and you are there.

FIRST CHOICE
Armed and Extremely Dangerous and The Player

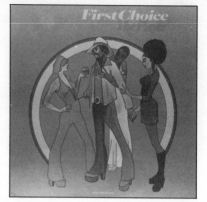

Philly Groove 1400 and 1502. "Girl groups" continued, with a wonderfully (stereo) typical trio whose sharp, sassy sound deserves a place up there with the greats of the Sixties. Prime assets: tight, drive-'em-up-the-walls production by Stan Watson and Norman Harris (Philadelphia again), hard vocals and rough and ready songs like "Armed and Extremely Dangerous," "Smarty Pants," "The Player"—all about being loved and left—"Newsy Neighbors" and a stunning version of Al Green's "Love and Happiness."

GLORIA GAYNOR
Never Can Say Goodbye and Experience

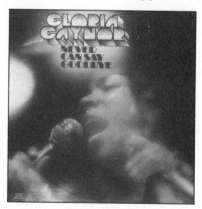

MGM M3G–4982 and M3G–4997. Gaynor is a "girl group" all by herself, a fine shouter with enough power to keep her head above some of the most ornate, overblown and totally arresting production numbers since disco was born. Her debut album was the first to put a disco mix of songs on record: "Honeybee," "Never Can Say Goodbye" and "Reach Out, I'll Be There" blended together a never-ending drumbeat, to make an almost 20-minute medley. The formula was repeated on the first side of the followup album, ending with a disco-style "How High the Moon." Both side twos are filler, but the overall format is a breakthrough for the disco market.

EDDIE KENDRICKS
People ... Hold On

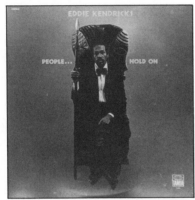

Tamia T315L. If there were no other cut on this album but "Girl You Need a Change of Mind," it would still deserve its status as one of the most important records in a disco library. "Girl," seven-and-a-half minutes long, is total: complex, dense, with a stirring production by Frank Wilson that never fails to bring screams from a dance floor. Also contains a minor gem, "Date with the Rain."

LOVE UNLIMITED
Under the Influence Of ...

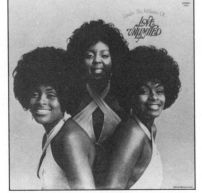

20th Century T–414. Another classic album, if only because of its opening cut, "Love's Theme," the instrumental that broke Barry White's Love Unlimited Orchestra in the discotheques. Like the rest, it's a spun-sugar composition thick with violins; lush enough to choke you, but irresistible. The vocals are vibrant and super sexy, the group at their best,

swathed in Barry White fantasies.

VAN McCOY
Disco Baby and The Disco Kid

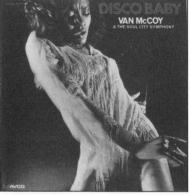

Avco AV69006–698 and AV-69009–698. McCoy's most successful record was "The Hustle," the record that accompanied 1975's major dance. It's the prime cut on *Disco Baby,* along with respectable instrumental versions of disco standards ("Doctor's Orders," "Fire," "Get Dancin' ") and excellent McCoy originals like the spicy "Spanish Boogie." *The Disco Kid* continues in the same mold, including a "Hustle" repeat called, predictably, "Keep on Hustlin'." McCoy is one of the key disco stylists (check out his work with Faith, Hope & Charity, David Ruffin and the Stylistics) and this is some of his best work.

GEORGE McCRAE
Rock Your Baby and
George McCrae

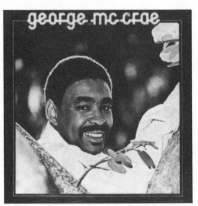

TK 501 and 602. The whole of McCrae's first album sounds like the title cut, but for those who swooned time after time to "Rock Your Baby" and its airy, float-away sound, there's nothing to complain about. Dance right through the nine songs—and the almost identical numbers on the followup LP—without losing the beat once.

One of the most imitated sounds in the disco repertoire. The musicians: KC & the Sunshine Band.

THE RITCHIE FAMILY
Brazil

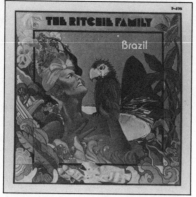

20th Century T–498. Lush, bright instrumental numbers by a batch of Sigma Sound musicians (MFSB by any other name) and a few female voices, sparked by the title cut and two other pop standards re-worked for disco dancers and blended together on the run-through first side. Most involving cut: "Frenesi," which is eight minutes long.

SILVER CONVENTION
Save Me

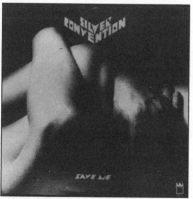

Midland International BKLI–1129. The European eclectic sound taken in another direction by a group living in Germany. The musicians are fronted by some sweet, ethereal female voices, which are mainly confined to simple chorus work over pretty, lightly choppy productions heavy on the strings. Not a lot of variety or content, but the mood is so consistently ecstatic and spacey it's as irresistible as a floor full of down cushions. "Fly, Robin, Fly," the album's longest cut, was one of 1975's major disco crossover records.

DONNA SUMMER
Love to Love You Baby

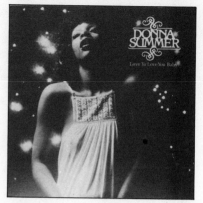

Oasis OCLP 5003. The album's title cut, filling up the entire first side and running nearly 17 minutes, is an erotic tour de force, more a production number than a mere song. Summer, an American living and recording in Germany, moans, purrs, seethes and sings what few lyrics there are with breathy abandon. The densely orchestrated production matches her passion, always on the verge of climax.

TRAMMPS

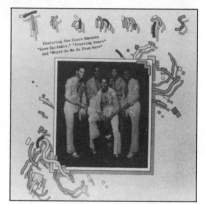

Golden Fleece KZ33163. Perhaps the definitive disco group, the Trammps continue to be especially popular in clubs because they haven't yet made the crucial crossover-to-pop move and risked being spoiled by exposure overground. And because they're one of the best male groups around. This album, their first, collects Trammps singles from the past few years, all produced by Ron Baker, Norman Harris and Earl Young, sharpest of the Philly B teams (Young is also a drummer/vocalist for the Trammps). Also pick up on the *Legendary Zing Album (Buddah BDS5641),* featuring the group's "Zing Went the Strings of My Heart."

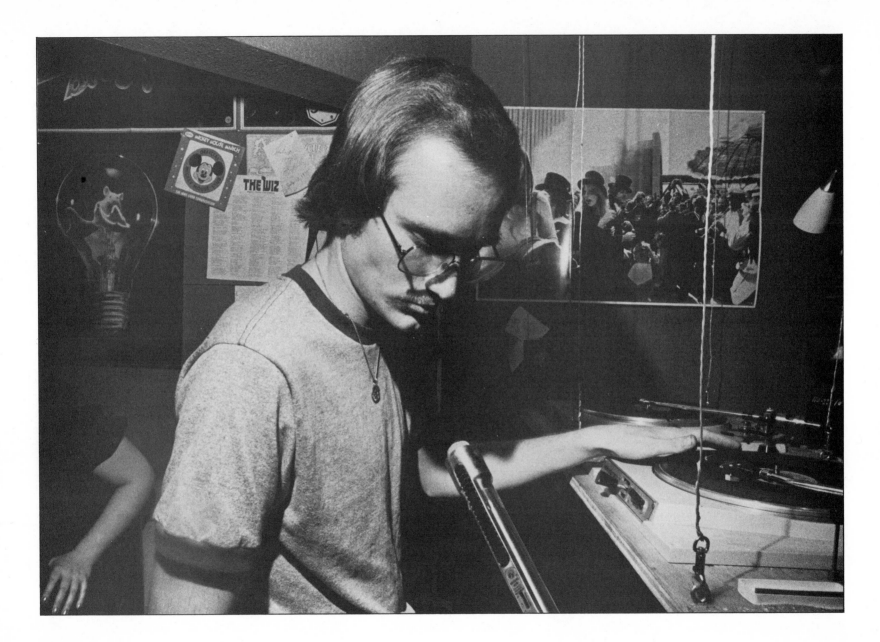

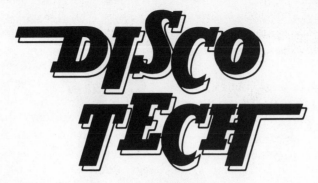

DISCO TECH

An All-American DJ Fights the Power
by Frank Robertson

The Chinese guy in a vest, no shirt, Levi's bellbottoms and his dancing partner, a white girl with a pert steno permanent and a red hot-pants suit, have obviously thought out a few things before taking to the disco floor. They look almost choreographed for the *Cher* show, except they probably wouldn't allow *this* on TV, the way he's arched backward on his hands and feet and she is straddling him, pumping down and up to the beat of "Fight the Power." The two gay black guys at the next table are checking this out and going "oooooowwwweeeeeeeee," as if this move is almost too cool to watch. Of course, not all the dancers are so explicit at the Dance Your Ass Off disco in North Beach, where 6500 predominantly straight, racially mixed dancers, mostly singles, show up each week and hustle the night away.

Dance Your Ass Off Inc., formerly an elite gay nightclub called Olympus, is two stories—about one-half acre—of funky couches, tables, stuffed chairs, two bars, a soon-to-be-completed restaurant and a dance floor over which hang four bass and four midrange red, white and blue 15-inch Altec speaker cabinets. Also above most of the scene is DJ Pete Struve, age 22, who sits in his second-story booth, surrounded by two floating QRK turntables, a Crown amp, a Russco mixer, a graphic equalizer, a board monitor, several stacks of 45s, shelves of LPs, a roll of toilet paper, light bulbs, a desk fan, a Motown "Disc-O-Tech" pennant, a tall Tom Collins and his Marlboros. Besides the audio show, Struve controls, with a battery of switches, the supporting cast of lights—five mirror balls, a Dance Your Ass Off sign that flashes on and off, Kinomatic projectors, the Powerstat theater dimmer and the strobe—and while he watches his board's VU needles bouncing to the beat of the music he selects and cues records. "You mix from one cut into the next and try to keep it popping," says Pete. "If it's just not doing it, I'll take it out, you know, and try something else. Of course there are guaranteed-to-get-'em-off-their-asses songs, like 'Shining Star,' 'Cut the Cake' or anything by the Isley Brothers, heh, heh.

"Every DJ does his own type of trip," Pete continues. "One of my favorite segues is from 'Shame, Shame, Shame' to 'Spirit of the Boogie.' Or you discover certain songs that go together, maybe spell out a thought in titles. Like one of my favorites is by Lynn Collins, 'Think about It'; I go into 'You're the One' by the Three Degrees, and out of that into 'Fight the Power' by the Isleys, and at the beginning of 'Fight the Power' I go, 'Hey, think about it 'cause you're the one, so fight the power.'

"I'm the only person I know of in town who plays slow music once in a while. They really like it. They get real, heh, heh, close and they do it, and that's cool. I think a lot of music that's coming out is kind of antipeople. Belligerent. Fighting-type music like 'Kung Fu Fighting,' which we blacklisted. 'Fight the Power' might be blacklisted soon, because it is, you know, kill-type music. I think instead of this kill-type music, let's use get-'em-up-type music."

Pete is not your glittery, androgynous type; under his glasses he looks a little like a fair-haired Roger Miller. He went to San Francisco's Bailey School of Broadcasting—he says his voice is lower now, and he's more confident using it. He'd like to be an FM DJ someday. At Dance Your Ass Off he announces records he thinks the dancers might not be familiar with, and when the mood hits, he works on his exhortations. "Bohannon's 'Foot-Stompin' Music,'" Pete notes, "has a part in it that says, 'If you feel like clappin' your hands, clap your hands.' So the song went on a ways and I went, 'If you feel like clappin' your hands, clap your hands!' And everybody's out there clap

clap clap. I said, 'I know the time is now! If you feel like screamin', scream!' And the whole place screamed. And I said, 'I can't hear ya!' And they screamed louder. I said, 'I can't hear ya!' They screamed louder, and I went, 'I hear ya now.'"

Whatever he may lack in hip Wolfman Jack charisma, Struve makes up for in his knowledge of and ideas for his tools. "Most disc jockeys know nothing about the equipment, except that turntables go around with records on them and you put the needle on the records," he says. "I have—I guess it's called a mechanical mind."

Struve came to Dance Your Ass Off as an audio-repair technician with ambitions to become a disco DJ. "I would look at the equipment, calibrate the turntables, balance the equalizer, maintain the system. One day I got a phone call saying, 'Hey, our DJ just quit. Are you ready? Grab your records.' And I went, 'Uh huh, here we go.' Heh, heh. So I got all threaded out and came in on a Saturday night with 1400 people in here."

Struve pulls out a drawing he's made of the new booth he has planned for Dance Your Ass Off which will have, in addition to what he's already got, a TEAC tape deck, Meteor Lighting equipment, new tweeters in the cabinets and a TV camera with pan, tilt and zoom, hooked up to a six-by-eight TV screen on the dance floor. "People can watch themselves boogieing on the floor. I'll be able to zoom in on anyone. And say I'm watching the *Midnight Special* on my monitor screen in front of me and I see the South Shore Commission or something coming up with 'Free Man' or a hot song and I go haaaaa! Chicachicachica—throw a couple of switches—not only will the people be listening to the music on the floor, they'll be watching the performers on the screen. It'll be," he says, "the wildest disc jockey booth, if not in the world, in the nation."

Around spring 1975, Struve started receiving his records directly from the record companies. He prefers playing LPs rather than 45s ("better quality"), listens to an average of 50 singles and albums a week and plays whatever he likes. "Honey Trippin' " by Mistic Moods is cued on the turntable and Struve flicks the button to turn it loose on the dancers. "This will go radio, definitely," he says, bending over to the Graphic equalizer and sliding the knobs up for more bass and drums. An equalizer will alter or "EQ" an amplifier so that certain frequencies are more or less pronounced than others; Struve uses his on everything, usually to bring out the lows on a record to strengthen, say, a weak or buried horn section.

"I was the first Bay Area person to play 'Giddyap Girl,' " says Struve, about the Bareback Rockers song that was produced by his main man and sent to Pete with a label saying "Bob Crewe presents for private stock records for disco DJs only!!!" "The single sounded terrible. I stacked it. I have a stack of records on the very top shelf, where I have trouble reaching, and those are the shit records. We get a lot of 'em. Then I got the Bob Crewe mix and I listened to it again, and it was fantastic. Really hot and strong. I started playing it a couple of days ago. It's gonna go. I mean a song, the first time they hear it, they pack the floor. It's good.

"You should see that whole dance floor full of people doing the Hustle. Everybody on the floor doing the Hustle at once. It's the most fantastic thing you've ever seen in your life. And then I'll put a record on just to break it up. Just to blow 'em away. Heh, heh." Pete plays "I'll Be Holding On" by Al Downing, and looks out on the floor. "They're all out there doing the L.A. Hustle," he says. He cues up "The Hustle" and grabs a chrome whistle attached to a key ring. "I just bought this today," he says. "Close your ears." He punches a button on the board to mix into "The Hustle" and blows the whistle into his microphone. He loves it.

Struve works as a DJ an average of four nights a week, usually Monday through Thursday, and he still does maintenance on the sound system and the lights. "Yeah, I change all the damn light bulbs, and we get new effects all the time. I'm putting them in, installing stuff, doing odd jobs off the wall.

"I'm getting $30 a night for spinning records. I know I should be earning almost twice that much, but I'm getting paid for being around and doing the lights and stuff, so it averages out. I'm having a good time. I don't need a lot of money to live on. I get a little upset once in a while, going home alone all the time but, you know, that'll cure itself in time. I mean, I've never been so happy in my life. This is it. I'm in heaven, heh, heh. I get high alone, just on playing records for people and seeing them dance."

And what does Pete the disco DJ listen to when the lights come up and everybody leaves?

"I go home and listen to classical."

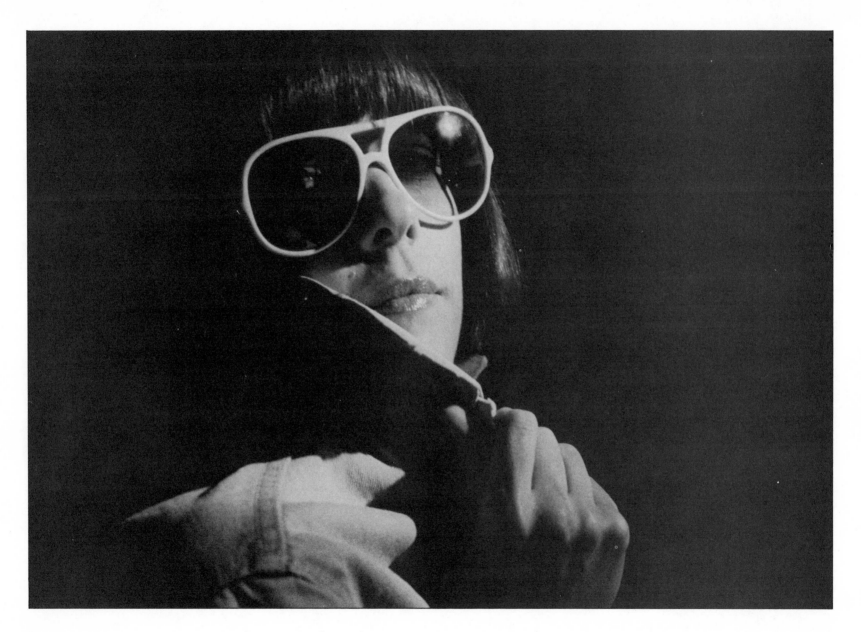

CONFESSIONS OF THE DISCO KID

A Woodstock Sun-Groper
Locks Hips with the Soviet Bulldozer
by Cindy McEhrlich

The Disco floor with the houselights up is about as glamorous as Ginger Rogers without makeup. But we were there to work, all 50 or so of us—swingles, out-patients, foreign students, dental hygienists—a forlorn and frightened group that wanted to emerge full-blown when the mirror balls sparkled and the magic began.

What had I gotten mixed up in? Nobody I knew learned to dance in a class, they just *did* it. This baleful group had been lured by the Sunday paper's pink section, billboards and tourist guides to learn an actual Dance Craze. At four bucks an hour, we would learn a new dance each week, for as long as the dances were devised. More important, really, we would perhaps capture The Disco Look.

Karen Lustgarten, our instructor, for sure had The Look. A balloon-sculpture body straight out of Archie and Veronica,

bright red hair and a kid-next-door face. She was like a friendly caricature, an image that rang bells in the past but was definitely new. She had the strut, the cocky swing and dip, that Disco is all about. And she got us all through the Bump, the Dinosaur and two versions of the Hustle by lying outrageously about how good we looked, demanding sweat and laughing along with us.

Arthur Murray's it was not. The dance floor in this off-hours Disco was conveniently adjacent to the bar, where most of the students tanked up before class. A low-key hysteria pervaded, a perpetual nervous laugh which kept everybody smiling. That, we were told, was the most important thing: "Keep smiling, no matter what."

I regarded my fellow students smugly. Obviously, many of them had cut their teeth on modern dance or the Woodstock

Sungrope. They'd either come off like Russ Tamblyn or be unable to manage a disciplined step to save their lives. I consoled myself that, no matter what, here was a group I could top.

I was wrong. I tried rationalizing: I was wearing deck shoes that wouldn't slide; my blouse was too tight; the people made me nervous; I needed a drink. But the truth is, I was stiff. I didn't have The Disco Feeling. I was doing the Stroll when I was supposed to be doing the Hustle. The nondescript admixture of steps I had developed through the light-show years wasn't working.

The L.A. Hustle is a quick ticket to the thrill of a chorus line. I don't want to get too mystical about it, but there's nothing quite like doing the same step at the same time as 50 other people, surging forward, backward and sideways as one. There's also nothing like being the only person going the wrong way in a roomful of unstoppable dancers, especially when they come to the kick.

But everybody's favorite dance—except mine—seemed to be the Bump, in which, ideally, you brush some portion of your body in a rhythmic way against some portion of your partner's body, gracefully swerving in the opposite direction on the off beat.

On the first night of Bump class I landed a Russian bulldozer as a partner. "Dis a wery sexy donce," he announced without smiling. Every time his Soviet hip plowed my way, I had visions of fly-

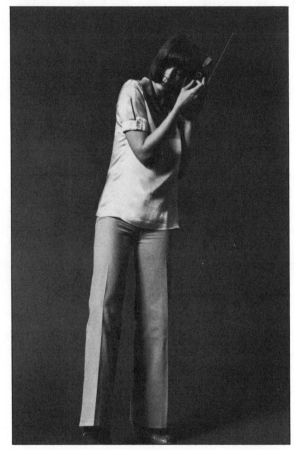

ing through the plate glass window—no doubt surprising the crowd which had gathered out on the sidewalk to laugh at us. I bumped back furiously, just to keep my footing.

Our coach had delicately omitted the extenuating possibilities of the Bump, centering our practice around ass, shoulder and knee bumping, but insisting that we vary them. The knee bump struck me as potentially lethal, and the Rusky must have seen the gleam in my eye. "Don't bompt vit your knee ven I face you," he warned me.

Then I got entangled with a Samoan swingle in a Wet-Look bodyshirt. This guy decided to skip the preliminaries; when the music started I was driven amongst the upholstered chairs by this maniac, thrusting pelvicly ever forward and wiggling his hands above his head like Bela Lugosi.

This kind of perverted Doris Day plot kept happening, partly because there is something really old-fashioned about Disco. Shades of the past are obvious in dances like the New York Hustle, which is done in Social Dance Position. When you're in Social Dance Position, you'd better chat or things get a little tense. They can get tense anyhow.

I don't recollect everyone being quite so *sweaty* in high school: My partner this time around managed to sponge up a respectable amount with my blouse when he put his hand on my waist. We had difficulty keeping our outstretched hands clasped because they were so slippery, but we made a brave show of teeth.

"I just walked in off the street," he said, a pretty self-demeaning thing to say, I thought. "We sail for Long Beach tomorrow." Trouble. Dear God, a sailor. My hand lightened on his shoulder. "Came down from Vancouver and Seattle this week ..." he began. This guy was on the verge of a travelogue. In that moment I understood the liberation of dances without partners—just as they were on the verge of going out of fashion.

Disco has brought back the Hangout, a place to go for a few hours that doesn't cost too much, where people dance or get smashed or just look cool. It's like an endless sock hop for post-teenagers, updated, of course, by tequila, amyl nitrate and a varying degree of pornography. Superflies, hobbits, dream queens, punks—the crowds are as democratic as they were in anybody's cafetorium.

Although the San Francisco discos open at nine, things don't really begin to pop until maybe 10:30. When I went to try my wings, we found an uncomfortably small crowd at opening time. The DJ screwed up his transitions and wiped out the dancers, clearing the floor with a too fast "Jumpin' Jack Flash." We burrowed into a couch. At 10:30, just as the music smoothed out and the floor started filling, in walked The Last Person in the World We Wanted to See. We dove behind the couch, crawled out the rear exit and hit the sack at 11:00.

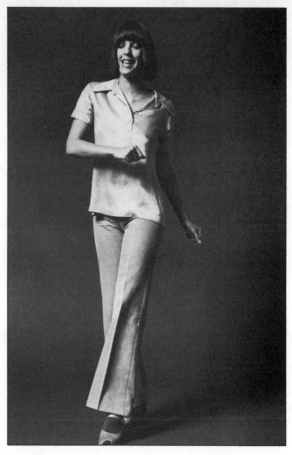

But my moment of glory finally came at a party last weekend. As I hung out near the stereo, someone recalled that I was learning Disco (after I yelled, "Where the fuck's the dancing?" a few times). Since I was sportily and quite by chance wearing a comfortable gym suit and tennies, I volunteered to give lessons. By the time I left, a dozen more people in this world knew the basics of the L.A. Hustle. But *my* stroke, as someone so acutely noticed, had That New Feeling. I had turned the corner from the Stroll.

Now I think Disco. Songs I used to think were boring, like "The Hustle," I like now because they're good to dance to. The groove is to dance for hours without stopping in a kind of alert stupor.

I've started correcting my stance in windows, snatching a few quick steps en route from the kitchen to the bedroom, working in a little shoulder action on the way to the bank. And I've stopped answering friends who watch and ask, "Doesn't it get boring?" Watching is not the point. Watching is boring.

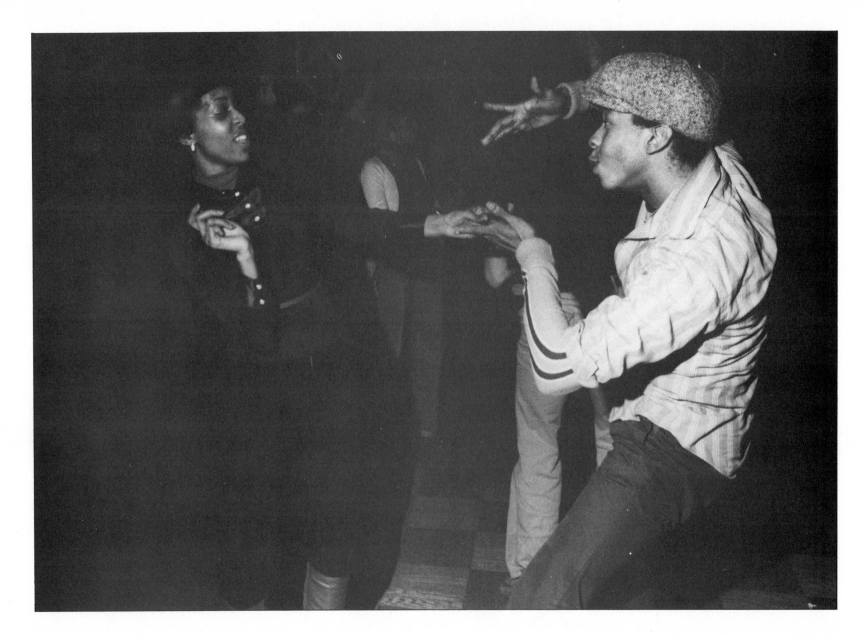

THE NEW YORK HUSTLE

At Last, a Perfect Anthem for the Five Boroughs
by Karen Lustgarten and Ralph Lew

The Hustle is the main "touch dance" of the Seventies. Hustlers dance it to the latest favorites and to disco standards like Van McCoy's "The Hustle" and the Ritchie Family's version of "Brazil." Since it became popular in late 1974, variations like the Continental Hustle and the Latin Hustle have nearly replaced the Basic New York Hustle as the latest rage on the disco scene.

About all the various versions have in common is that they are done with a partner in the Social Dance Position and involve intricate turns which give the dances their distinctive flow and beauty. The Social Dance Position may have been before your time: The man and woman (or any modern combination) face each other, the woman's left hand resting on the man's upper arm, the man's right hand on her waist. Their other hands are extended to the side and clasped. This is just the starting point, but the constant factor will be that at least one hand is to remain clasped with your partner's.

A basic New York Hustle has a step-tap-step-tap pattern. On the first count of the music, the man steps about eight inches to the left with his left foot. Then he takes step two, tapping his right foot next to his left so his heels form a T. For step three, the man steps to his right with his right foot, and he completes the pattern by tapping his left foot to his right so that his heels form another T. Each step takes the same amount of time; take small steps, since the music is usually fast and you won't make the pattern if you're too slow.

35

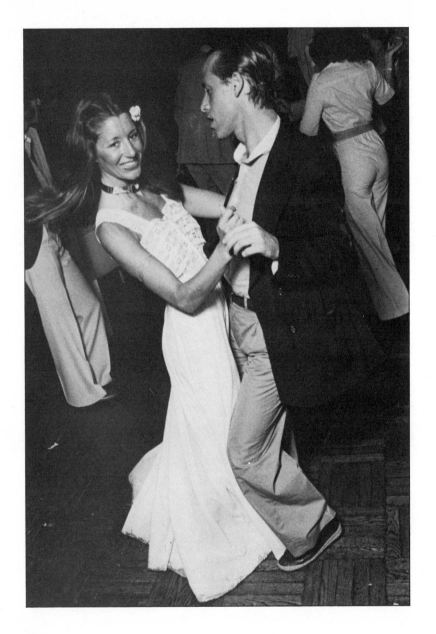

That's one pattern. The directions should be reversed for the woman (i.e., right, left, left, right) since she and her partner have to move in the same direction.

Though the above version of the Hustle is done in four counts, most Hustles are done in six. The Continental (also called the American) adds two steps to the basic pattern, with each step equaling one count. The last two steps are forward in the first part, backward in the next. Again, the woman's directions are reversed.

The Latin Hustle is more complex. It's danced to six beats, but it includes seven steps; two of them (count "three-and") equal one beat. On count one the man taps his left foot to his right foot. Then, on count two, he steps to the left side with his left foot. For "three-and" he crosses his right foot in back of his left, landing on the ball as he makes a quarter turn to the right, and then skips back so his left foot meets the right. (The man may drop his right hand, the woman her left.) On count four he steps forward with his right foot, on count five forward with his left, and on six he steps forward with the right and turns again to face his partner. The woman does the reverse steps, the partners repeat their patterns.

The following charts should help you master our basic step and the Continental and Latin Hustles. We've also included a variation of the Latin Hustle; eight steps done within six beats. When you have a pattern down, fan the pages and follow Robert Grossman's Hustle All-Stars through their turns. They take three steps to complete, and it's best to start on the third count.

Hurry up now: It's time to do the Hustle!

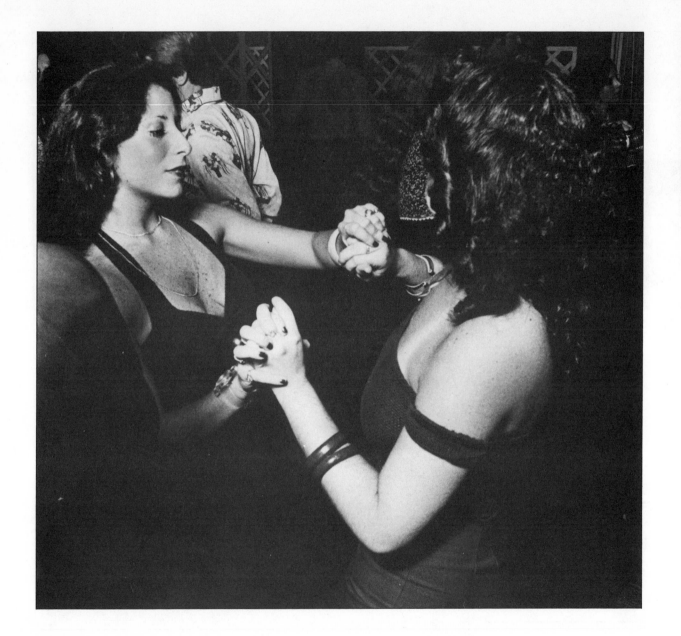

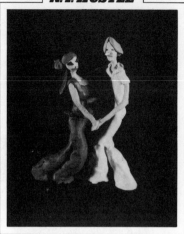

1) Loosen up by getting in the Social Dance Position and rocking toward your extended hands.

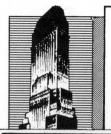

The New York Hustle

COUNTS	1	2	3	4	1	2	3	4
MAN'S FEET	STEP L	TAP R	STEP R	TAP L	STEP L	TAP R	STEP R	TAP L
WHERE	TO LEFT	TO L FOOT	TO RIGHT	TO R FOOT	TO LEFT	TO L FOOT	TO RIGHT	TO R FOOT
RHYTHM		ACCENT		ACCENT		ACCENT		ACCENT
WOMAN'S FEET	R	L	L	R	R	L	L	R

The Continental Hustle

COUNTS	1	2	3	4	5	6
MAN'S FEET	STEP L	TAP R	STEP R	TAP L	STEP L	STEP R
WHERE	TO LEFT	TO L FOOT	TO RIGHT	TO R FOOT	FWD (OR BKWD)	FWD (OR BKWD)
RHYTHM		ACCENT		ACCENT		
WOMAN'S FEET	R	L	L	R	R	L

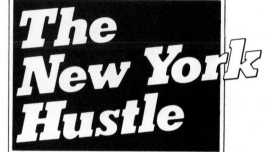

BASIC

COUNTS	1	2	3	AND	4	5	6
MAN'S FEET	TAP L	STEP L	STEP R	STEP L	STEP R	STEP L	STEP R
WHERE	TO R FOOT	TO LEFT	CROSS BACK OF L FOOT (¼ TURN TO RIGHT)	BACK TO R FOOT	FWD	FWD	TURN TO FACE PARTNER
RHYTHM			QUICK	QUICK			
WOMAN'S FEET	R	R	L	R	L	R	L

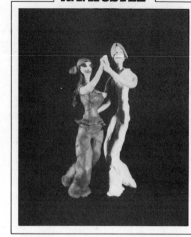

N.Y. HUSTLE

2) Rock back for the second triplet.

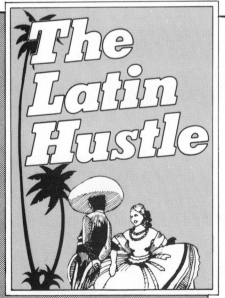

The Latin Hustle

VARIATION

COUNTS	1	2	3	AND	4	AND	5	6
MAN'S FEET	TAP L	STEP L	STEP R	STEP L	KICK R	STEP R	STEP L	STEP R
WHERE	TO R FOOT	TO LEFT	CROSS BACK OF L FOOT (¼ TURN TO RIGHT)	BACK TO R FOOT	SLIGHTLY WITH KNEE BENT	IN PLACE	FWD	TURN TO FACE PARTNER
RHYTHM			QUICK	QUICK	QUICK	QUICK		
WOMAN'S FEET	R	R	L	R	L	L	R	L

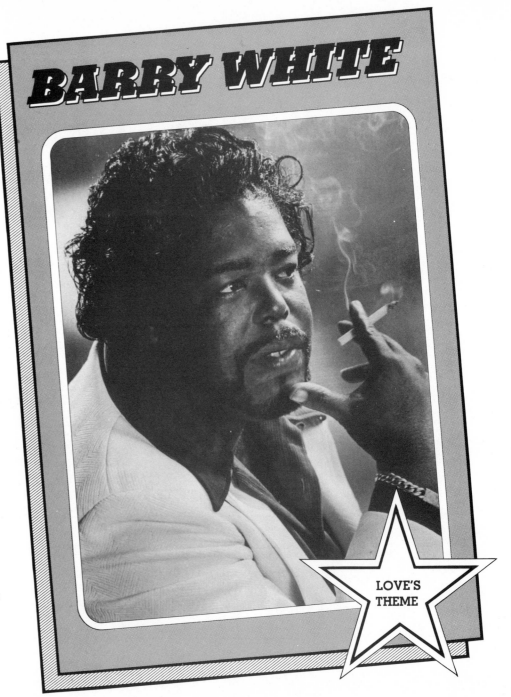

BARRY WHITE

BARRY WHITE

Responsible for much of the strings and lushness attributed to disco, White's "Love's Theme," "You're the First, the Last, My Everything" and "What Am I Gonna Do with You" merged ambitious arrangements with Barry's lover-boy growl.

As successful onstage as in the studio, Barry has toured the U.S. and Europe with his Love Unlimited Orchestra and three Love Unlimited backup singers. Critics put him down; his fans go wild.

White's sweeping, stylized arrangements combine strings and horns with a modicum of funk. Lyrically, Barry sings about love, and effectively merges emotion with rhythm to produce an instantly recognizable sound.

LOVE'S
THEME

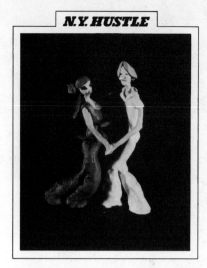

N.Y. HUSTLE

3) Try it again. Rock toward your hands . . .

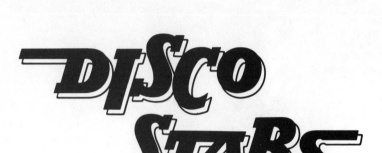

DISCO STARS

**_Their Secrets Revealed...Hustle Wit...
Bunny's Hop... Is This Liberation?...Evolution?...Fad?...
God Only Knows...It's All Greek to Us...
by Tom Vickers_**

KC AND THE SUNSHINE BAND

H. W. Casey and Rick Finch, leaders of the Sunshine Band, worked in the warehouse at TK Records before their trademark disco sound won them success both in England and the States. Instead of relying on Arps, synthesizers and other electronic gadgetry, KC produced effects with normal instruments. "Get Down Tonight," with its speeded up guitar intro and horn-punctuated "Do a little dance/Make a little love/Get down tonight" refrain was an example of the group's warm, optimistic sound, as was the followup, "(That's the Way) I Like It."

Unlike many voguish producers, Casey (seated 5th from left) doesn't specifically work toward disco play. "My approach is based on just how it sounds to me. I cut a record to sound the way I want it to sound. Sounds come out of knowing what's right. I feel everything I do."

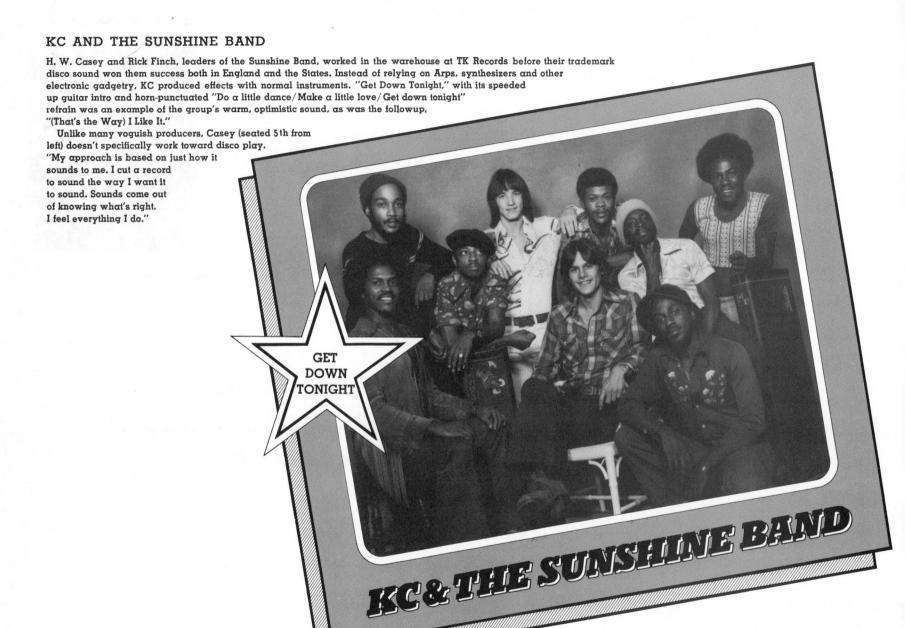

GET DOWN TONIGHT

KC & THE SUNSHINE BAND

VAN McCOY

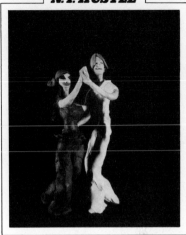

4) Good. Now rock back and get ready to release the shoulder and waist hands. You're about to try a turn, keeping your extended hands together.

VAN McCOY

The Hustle Man has been in the music business for more than a dozen years, originally as a songwriter, then as producer, arranger and performer (piano and backup vocals). Though his 'Disco Baby' and 'Disco Kid' albums offered the backbeat, strings and chorus associated with mainstream disco music, they weren't drastically different from the middle-of-the-road material he recorded with Mitch Miller in 1966. If the Miller album was "easy listening," 'Disco Kid' was "easy dancing."

McCoy heard about the Hustle from a disc jockey at New York's Adam's Apple, but claims that he never saw it danced until after he recorded his namesake single. McCoy feels that the Hustle is different from other disco steps. "It's an intricate dance. It's more of a ballroom dance than a disco-Bump thing. There's so much diversification going on that it brings back partner dancing. There's always room for something new and good."

★ THE HUSTLE

43

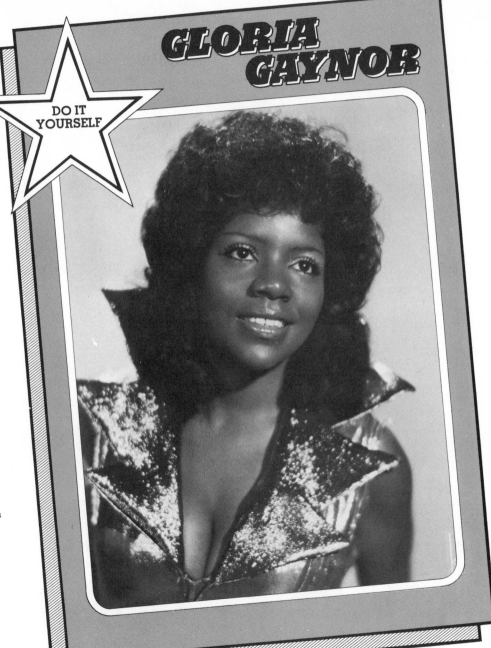

GLORIA GAYNOR

DO IT YOURSELF

GLORIA GAYNOR

Crowned Queen of the Discos at New York's Le Jardin, Gaynor is best known for her upbeat rendition of the Jackson 5's "Never Can Say Goodbye." "Goodbye" and her later single, "How High the Moon"/"Do It Yourself," featured long, strong rhythm tracks that successfully held her wailing, undistinguished voice over a near orchestral mix.

Gaynor calls disco "happy music. It's a very good vehicle to get across anything you want to say, whether about love, politics or a message. People listen while they're dancing. I think it's the most diversified music going."

The Three Degrees, Esther Phillips and even David Bowie have challenged Gaynor's royal disco title, but she seems unconcerned. "Someone could be right on my heels. I don't follow the charts, so I don't really know."

FAITH HOPE & CHARITY

Working with producer Van McCoy, Diane Destry, Albert Bailey and Brenda Hilliard scored in the discos with "To Each His Own," which mixed their soaring ensemble vocals with McCoy's glossy, orchestrated production.

Singer Albert Bailey feels that disco is more than a fad. "I was in a disco last weekend and I've never seen a group of people so into the music." Destry sees the key to disco's success in the DJ. "He has to know what the various records are about and then have the ability to blend discs, to build a constant upper."

44

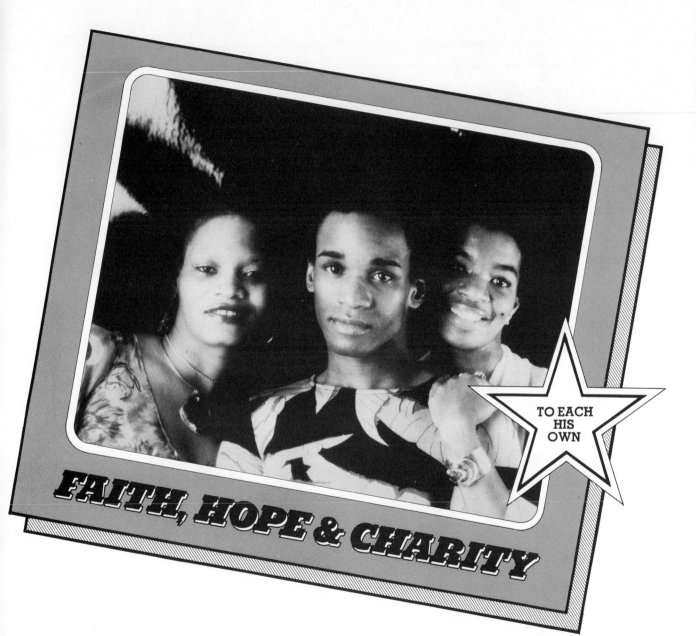

FAITH, HOPE & CHARITY

TO EACH
HIS
OWN

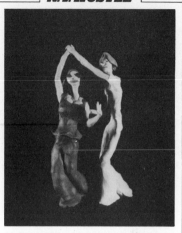

5) To turn, the man lifts his left arm for the woman to pass under.

OHIO PLAYERS

More than any other group, the Players have come to symbolize the most danceable elements of disco: a repetitious beat and howling vocals. Clarence Satchell (kneeling, glasses), the Players' reedman, sees disco as a continuation of earlier styles. "I think the people were dancing all along. We went through a period when we had mind and body dances. Then recently we had the Bump, symbolic of an era when dances were easy and anybody could do them. Now the disco thing may turn into the ballroom thing—who knows? Discos belong to the people.   The public invented it, and now business has capitalized on it." The Players' 'Honey' album contained mostly ballads; 1974's "Fire," with its screaming sirens and thundering backbeat, was a disco smash.

Satchell feels that discos will help make performing groups more popular. "The entertainer has replaced the movie star. People are always curious about their favorite acts and how they do their material."

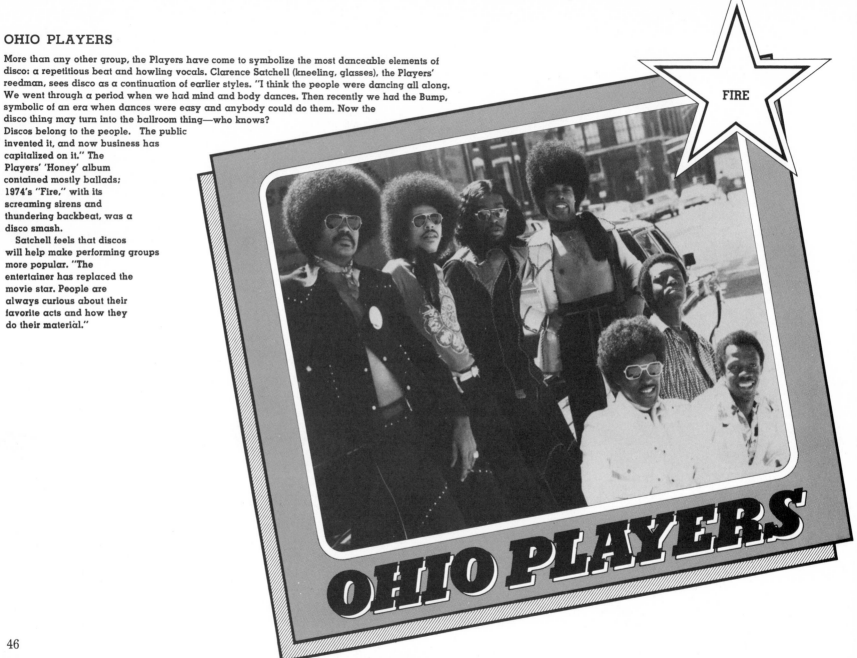

FIRE

OHIO PLAYERS

THE ISLEY BROTHERS

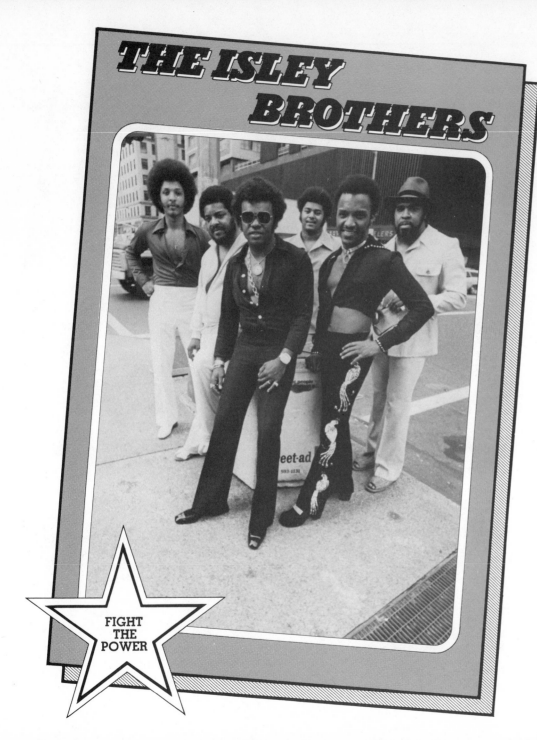

FIGHT
THE
POWER

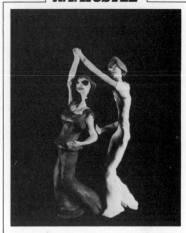

6) The woman has, miraculously, passed under!

THE ISLEY BROTHERS

Since late 1971, the Isleys have come on strong to the disco sound. "That Lady" was the harbinger of Isley hits like "Live It Up" and "Fight the Power." Their basic sound depends on a bass-dominated rhythm punctuated by enthusiastic vocals and brother Ernie's soaring, Hendrix-styled guitar. Ronald Isley (in front), the group's lead singer, explained the rise of discos in racial terms. "Black music has always been confined in some corner and when you confine music that people enjoy, it has to have an outlet. That's where you'll come up with the discotheque. The discos put the other [white] music in a corner." Ernie, the drum- and guitar-playing Isley, added, "The disco craze is getting a lot of attention right now, but all it means is that rock & roll is going back to what its original concept was supposed to be."

47

B.T. EXPRESS

Following 1974's churning "Do It" with the equally seductive "Express," B.T.'s R&B-like bass-line/falsetto-chorus sound continued in "Peace Pipe." Bill Risbrook (3rd from right), sax player with the six-man, one-woman (sultry-voiced Barbara Joyce) band, acknowledged that "discos are great for new artists who need exposure. Older artists get their records played automatically, whether it's good or not, but if you're a new group it's virtually impossible to be heard on the radio. If a record is going to hit, it's gonna hit first in the discos."

Risbrook disagrees with those who complain that disco music is monotonous. "The days of just having a beat are over. Things have to be put together musically to form a quality product."

PEACE PIPE

B.T. EXPRESS

BLACKBYRDS

WALKING
IN
RHYTHM

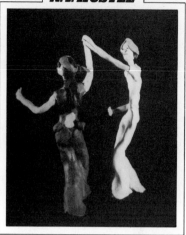

7) The woman continues her turn . . .

BLACKBYRDS

Trumpeter/former Howard University jazz teacher Donald Byrd formed the Blackbyrds in 1972, fulfilling his desire to head a group of high-caliber student musicians. They hit with the jazzy funk of "Walking in Rhythm," both on the radio and in the discos, and were heard in the movie 'Cornbread, Earl and Me.' Kevin Toney (top row center), keyboard player for the six-man group, sees discos "as a move you could expect. Disco reflects the economy and the fact that people want more out of a record—they want to dance and listen at the same time. Today's music is participatory music, the audience is just as much a part of the music as the musician."

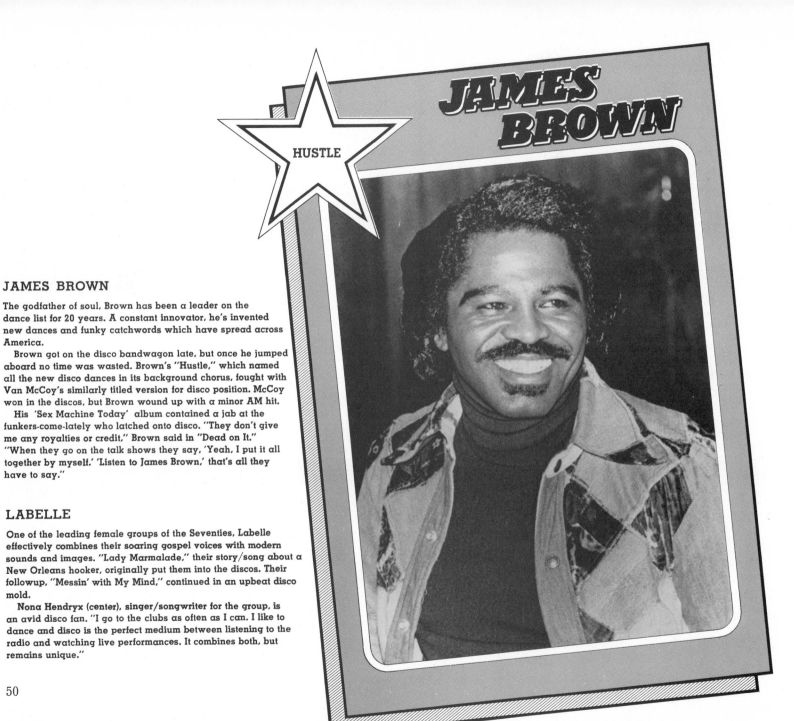

HUSTLE

JAMES BROWN

JAMES BROWN

The godfather of soul, Brown has been a leader on the dance list for 20 years. A constant innovator, he's invented new dances and funky catchwords which have spread across America.

Brown got on the disco bandwagon late, but once he jumped aboard no time was wasted. Brown's "Hustle," which named all the new disco dances in its background chorus, fought with Van McCoy's similarly titled version for disco position. McCoy won in the discos, but Brown wound up with a minor AM hit.

His 'Sex Machine Today' album contained a jab at the funkers-come-lately who latched onto disco. "They don't give me any royalties or credit," Brown said in "Dead on It." "When they go on the talk shows they say, 'Yeah, I put it all together by myself.' 'Listen to James Brown,' that's all they have to say."

LABELLE

One of the leading female groups of the Seventies, Labelle effectively combines their soaring gospel voices with modern sounds and images. "Lady Marmalade," their story/song about a New Orleans hooker, originally put them into the discos. Their followup, "Messin' with My Mind," continued in an upbeat disco mold.

Nona Hendryx (center), singer/songwriter for the group, is an avid disco fan. "I go to the clubs as often as I can. I like to dance and disco is the perfect medium between listening to the radio and watching live performances. It combines both, but remains unique."

50

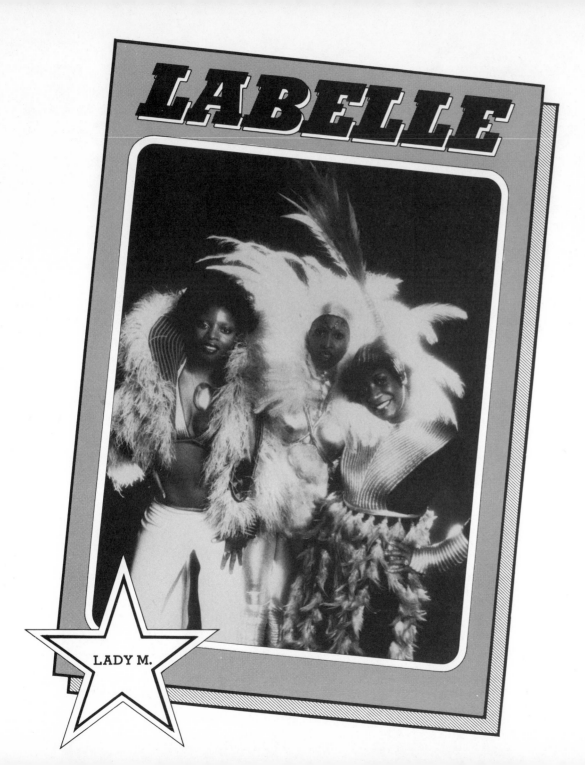

LABELLE

LADY M.

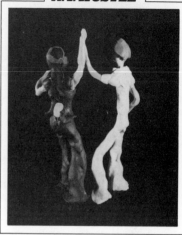

8) . . . until she faces her partner once again. The man has continued dancing in basic steps while she has been turning, so the dynamic duo is again moving from side to side in unison.

Those with vivid imaginations will realize that either of you can do the turn.

When the turn is completed, you can return to steps one to four. Or you can go have a drink.

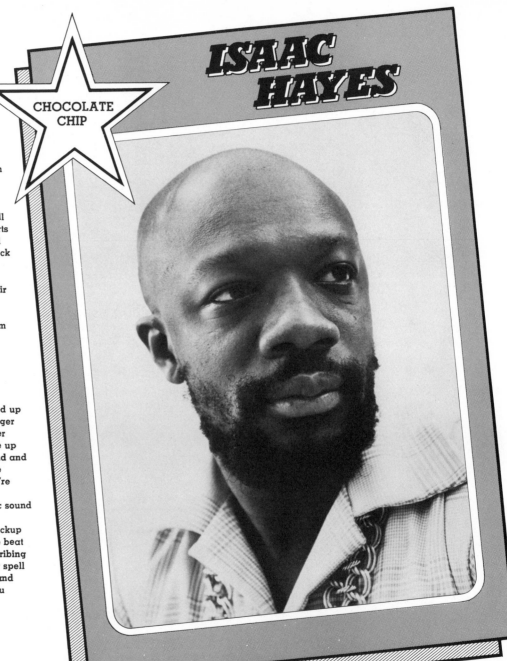

ISAAC
HAYES

CHOCOLATE
CHIP

ISAAC HAYES

This self-taught but remarkably resourceful arranger can make an electric bass line sound like it's being played by a section of tubas. The secret: He doubles it with an electric clavinet, then mixes the clavinet down into the track. "I depend on bass lines a lot," he said. "I write all of my bass lines out. I explain most of the rest of the parts by humming them to the musicians, including string and horn parts which I hum to an orchestrator, and then check when they're being recorded to be sure they're played right."

The 'Shaft' and 'Truck Turner' movie themes, with their simple drum patterns, topping congas, heavy bass and swirling orchestral overlays, were tailor-made for disco dancing: "Chocolate Chip" juxtaposed monolithic rhythm and trebly sweetening and was a disco chip off the old block.

THE RITCHIE FAMILY

Two Parisians, Henry Belolo and Jacques Morali, teamed up with group namesake and independent producer/arranger Richard Rome to produce "Brazil," a reworking of Xavier Cugat's Forties hit. Rome said that his two cohorts came up with an approach "somewhere between the Philly sound and Barry White, with strong rhythm, brass and strings." He elaborated: "We're trying to create our own sound. We're taking older big-band arrangements and putting them together with the disco sound. The result is a symphonic sound with disco soul rhythm."

In actuality, the Family is a group of Philadelphia backup singers and studio musicians assembled by Rome. "The beat should continue to build," the producer explained, describing his producing method, "but there should be a breathing spell with the orchestra. What I do is take out the orchestra and push the drums up in the mix. You can never relent. You never stop the beat once you start, but let it breathe in the middle."

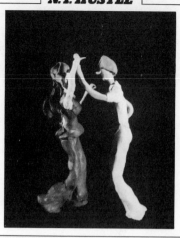

N.Y. HUSTLE

9) Onward to another turn where you go under each other's arm at the same time. Raise your extended arms and release your other set of hands.

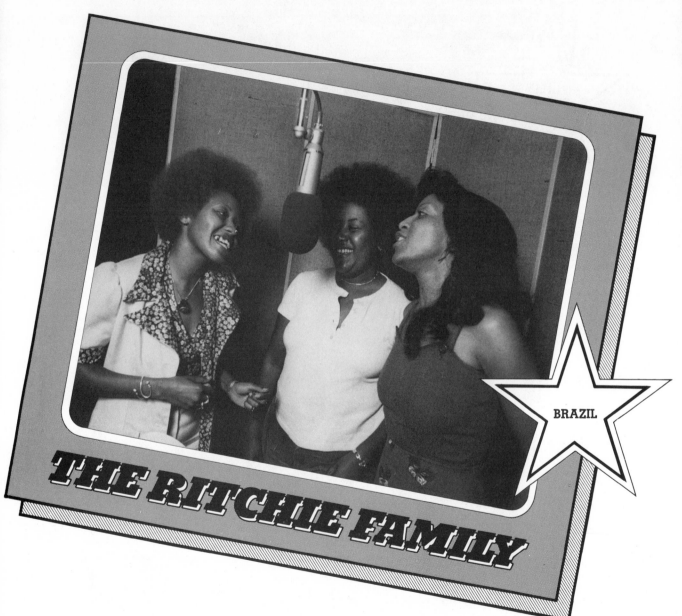

THE RITCHIE FAMILY

BRAZIL

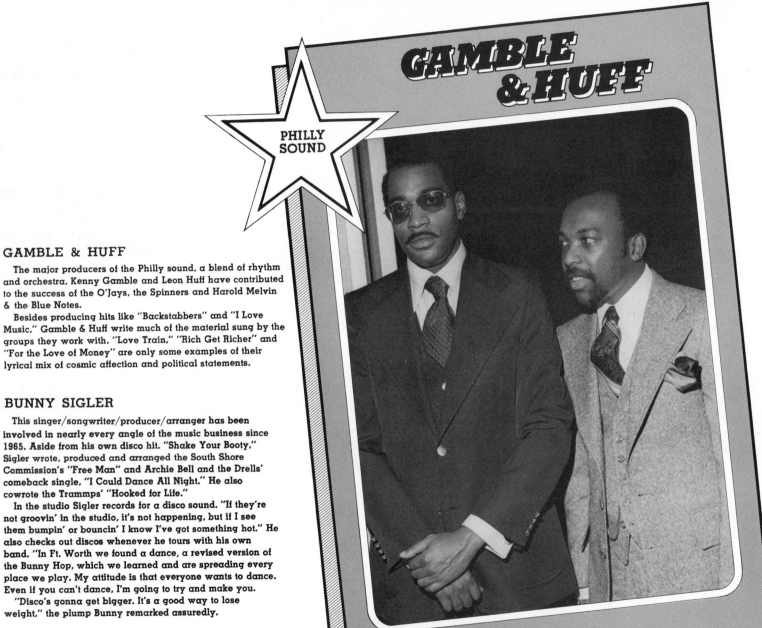

GAMBLE & HUFF

GAMBLE & HUFF

The major producers of the Philly sound, a blend of rhythm and orchestra, Kenny Gamble and Leon Huff have contributed to the success of the O'Jays, the Spinners and Harold Melvin & the Blue Notes.

Besides producing hits like "Backstabbers" and "I Love Music," Gamble & Huff write much of the material sung by the groups they work with. "Love Train," "Rich Get Richer" and "For the Love of Money" are only some examples of their lyrical mix of cosmic affection and political statements.

BUNNY SIGLER

This singer/songwriter/producer/arranger has been involved in nearly every angle of the music business since 1965. Aside from his own disco hit. "Shake Your Booty," Sigler wrote, produced and arranged the South Shore Commission's "Free Man" and Archie Bell and the Drells' comeback single, "I Could Dance All Night." He also cowrote the Trammps' "Hooked for Life."

In the studio Sigler records for a disco sound. "If they're not groovin' in the studio, it's not happening, but if I see them bumpin' or bouncin' I know I've got something hot." He also checks out discos whenever he tours with his own band. "In Ft. Worth we found a dance, a revised version of the Bunny Hop, which we learned and are spreading every place we play. My attitude is that everyone wants to dance. Even if you can't dance, I'm going to try and make you.

"Disco's gonna get bigger. It's a good way to lose weight," the plump Bunny remarked assuredly.

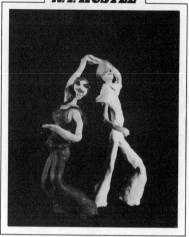

10) . . . allowing you both to go under

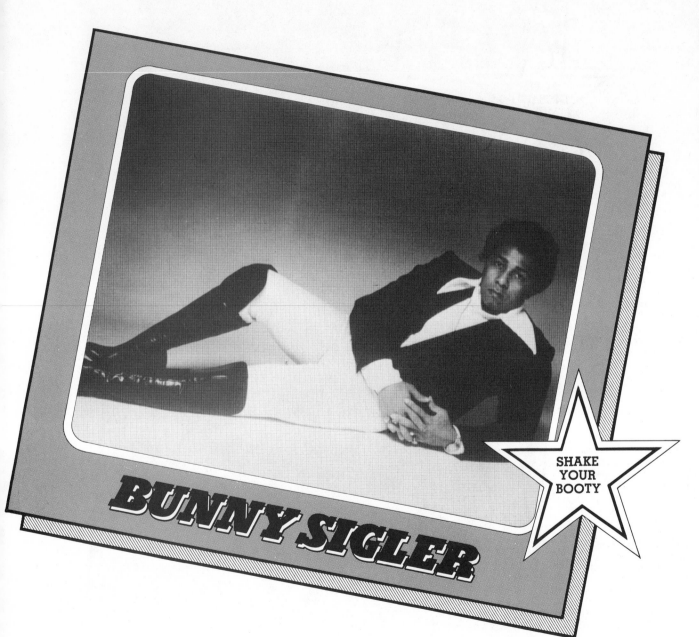

BUNNY SIGLER

SHAKE
YOUR
BOOTY

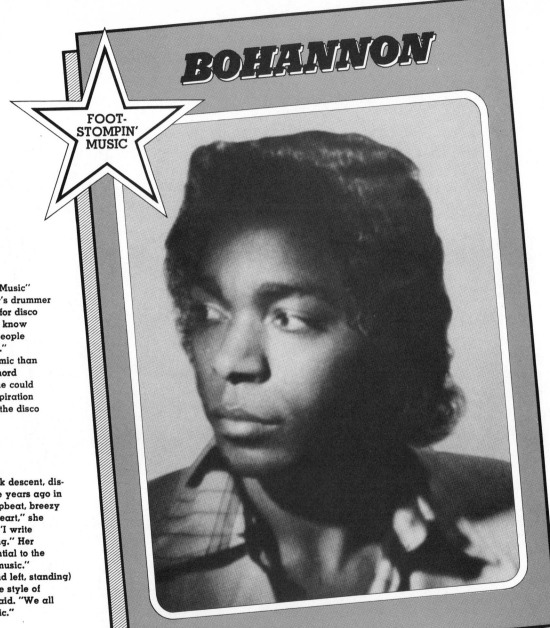

BOHANNON

FOOT-STOMPIN' MUSIC

BOHANNON

Known only by his last name to "Foot-Stompin' Music" fans, Bohannon's background as Stevie Wonder's drummer and a Motown bandleader left him ill-prepared for disco success. "When I first started recording, I didn't know anything about disco. I wanted to write music people could clap their hands and snap their fingers to."

His music is now more syncopated and rhythmic than when he was with Motown, but it has so few chord changes that Bohannon has half bragged that he could do an album a day. Bohannon feels that his inspiration "comes from God"; what the Lord thinks about the disco scene remains unknown.

CROWN HEIGHTS AFFAIR

Frieda Nerangis, a Brooklyn housewife of Greek descent, discovered this eight-member group in Harlem five years ago in 1970. Though she wrote the few words to the upbeat, breezy "Dreaming a Dream" and "Every Beat of My Heart," she doesn't write music. The secret of her success: "I write Greek and that helps me punctuate the phrasing." Her influence is felt in other ways. "I'm very influential to the guys as a female. I bring mellowness into the music."

Like Bohannon, bass player Muki Wilson (2nd left, standing) defines his music in religious terms. "Our whole style of playing is for people to clap their hands," he said. "We all believe in God and that comes over in our music."

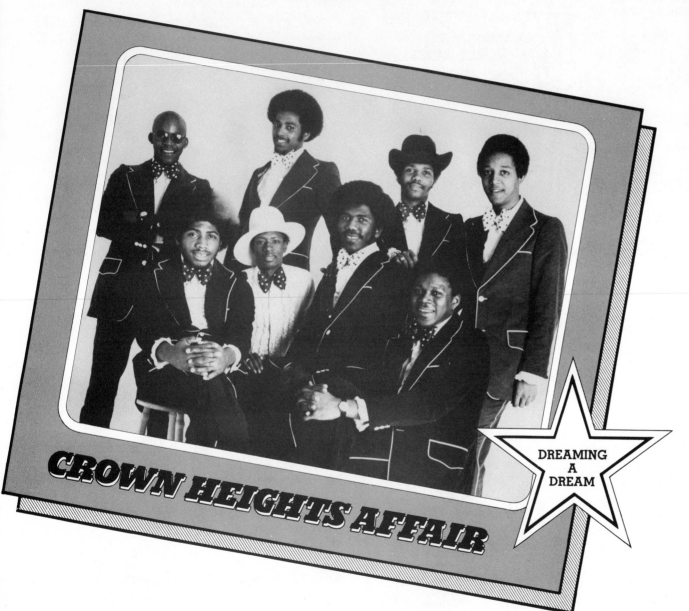

CROWN HEIGHTS AFFAIR

DREAMING A DREAM

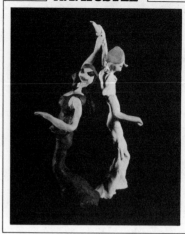

11) . . . rotating until each of you faces outward . . .

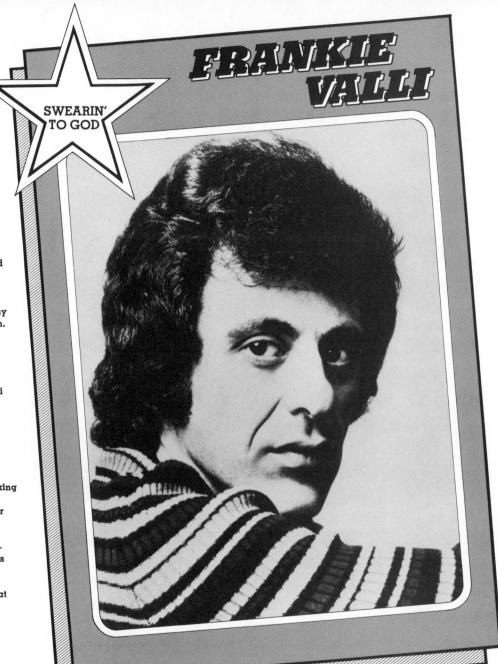

SWEARIN' TO GOD

FRANKIE VALLI

FRANKIE VALLI

The former Four Season (winter) made the disco charts with the crooning "Swearin' to God"—and immediately confessed that his hit was created with the discos in mind. The song made the pop charts, and Valli's tour featured some disco arrangements.

Valli's approach is straight MOR. "Some have criticized my show as being light, but it is designed for people to have fun. Why are we so geared to tragedy? Why not have fun?"

THE LOCKERS

Popular TV guests since choreographer/troupe member Toni Basil arranged for them to appear on a 1972 Roberta Flack special, the Lockers are best known for their outrageous costumes, story numbers like "Red Riding Hat" and, most of all, some high-energy dancing.

Group leader Don Campbell (in the striped vest) began to experiment with dancing in the late Sixties. He discovered that flapping his elbows, kicking out a knee, thrusting back with the opposite hip, rolling his wrist and pointing and locking every four beats was an effective cover for not being able to do the Funky Chicken. He called his dance the Lock. After becoming a regular on 'Soul Train,' he learned that dancing was "worth money."

Campbell's disco dancing involves a good deal of improvisation. "Even when I make a mistake like dropping my keys on the floor, I'll build my dance around picking them up. In fact, the dance is full of accidents."

Still, he sees dancing as "a competitive trip. I stopped in at the Destiny II," he said happily about a visit to a West L.A. club, "and t her dancers looked upset. They started thinking about second place."

THE LOCKERS

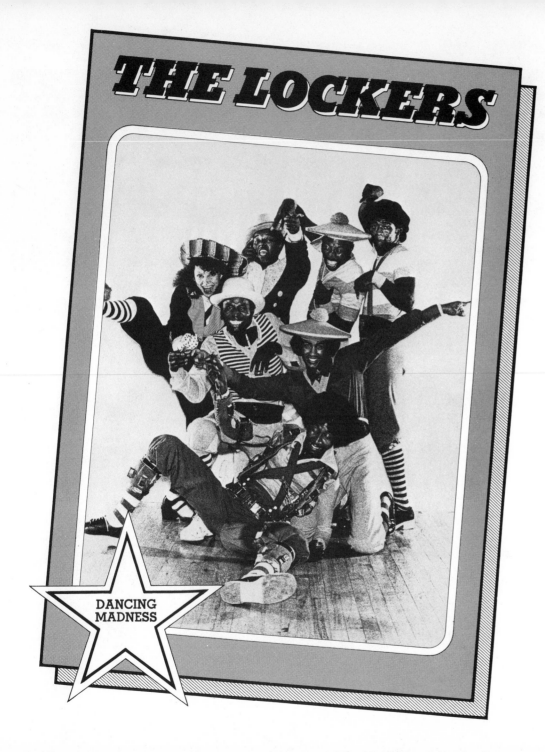

DANCING MADNESS

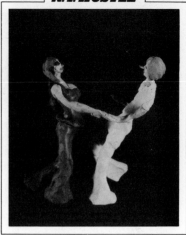

12) . . . and continuing around to a facing position.

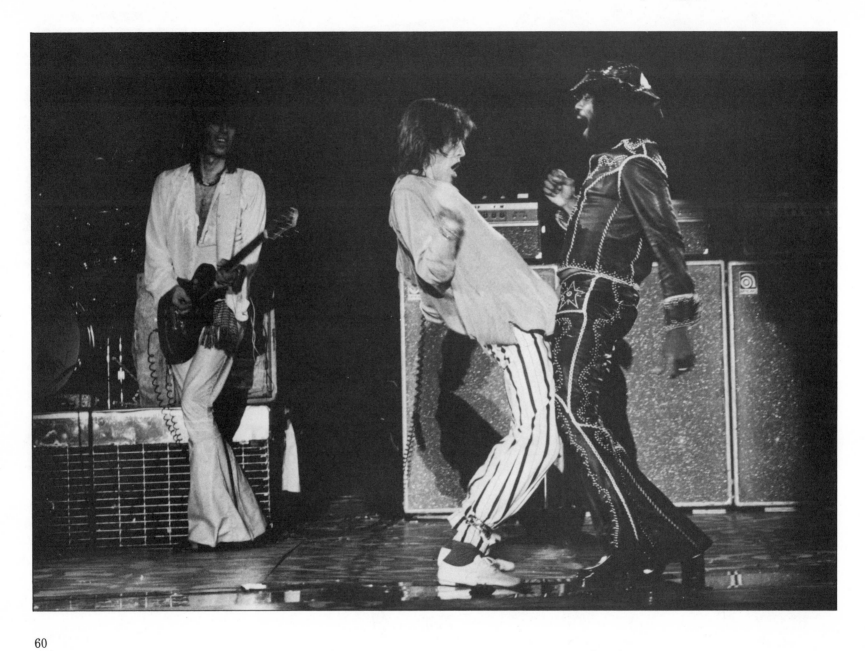

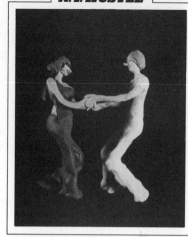

THE BUMP

What Has Four Hips and Grinds?

13) A snazzy variation is to keep hold of both pairs of hands, raise arms and do a double turn under them without letting go. This may land one of you in the hospital with a dislocated shoulder, so it might be time . . .

Although already obsolete in some parts of the United States, the Bump remains the best-known disco dance. This is probably because it's the easiest (and some say the most fun) dance to do. Just listen for a simple beat (as in the Isley Brothers' "Fight the Power") and remember that this dance is hip if your hips are good.

The Bump is done in multiples of two or four counts. The idea is to bump against your partner on the on beat and swing away for the off beat. If you bump twice in and twice out, you're doing the Double Bump; bump on every beat and you've transformed it into the Electric Bump.

There are no "steps": The feet are comfortably separated and pretty stationary, except when you need to move them to turn or keep your balance. The knees should be bent, the parts of the body not bumping should swing in the opposite direction from the part that's bumping, the whole body should be loose as a goose and it helps to be drunk. Only by coincidence should you be bumping with the same thing your partner bumps with, but for the sake of simplicity we've begun this sequence with both partners bumping the same thing in unison.—K.L.

61

Keep on Bumpin'

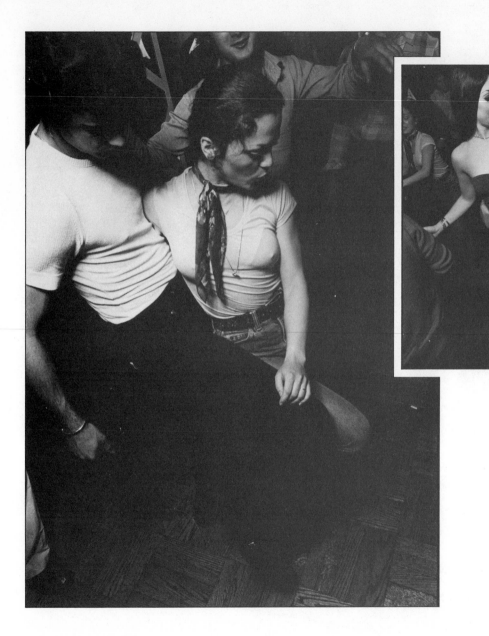

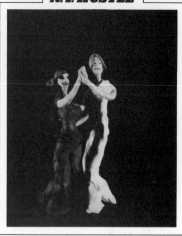

14) . . . for a peaceful interlude. Keep up the basic steps, rocking subtly from side to side and wondering what to do next.

1) Okay, let's begin with hip bumping. With knees slightly bent, bump hips, swinging arms and torso away from your partner.

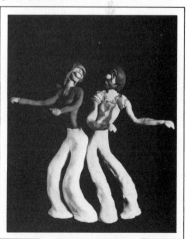

THE BUMP

THE KAY GEES

Beginning in 1972 as a high-school rhythm section in New Jersey, the Kay Gees added members gradually until the present seven-person unit jelled. Kevin Bell, younger brother of Kool and the Gang's Robert and Ronald Bell, produced their first hit, "Keep on Bumpin'," and the group's mixture of Arps, synthesizers and a strong backbeat were heard on "Hustle wit' Every Muscle."

Dennis White (middle row center), who plays tenor sax and flute with the group, was voted Prep Athlete of the year by 'Coach and Athlete' magazine for his achievements as a track star. White sees discos as an age phenomenon. "Now that people can drink at 18 in most states, there's no denial or fear to go out to a disco."

The Kay Gees are a straight-ahead disco group, though White feels that "discos definitely hurt live performances. People don't accept it as a show. You could be a record for all it matters."

KOOL AND THE GANG

One of the earliest and most important disco groups, their early hits, "Jungle Boogie," "Funky Stuff" and the whistle-blowing "Hollywood Singing," featured a crisp horn sound and telling Arp techniques. Their 1975 "Spirit of the Boogie" altered Kool's syncopated sound, depending more on vocals and chanted chorus than on instrumentation.

Robert "Kool" Bell (center) shies away from the disco label his group has attracted. "Our music is basic, energetic. We're not geared to one way. Being disco is fine, but being accepted in other forms of music is also important. The uptempo songs are getting stronger and stronger, to the point where the whole disco market is uptempo. I like to keep a balance, so we try to include some ballads and more relaxed stuff."

64

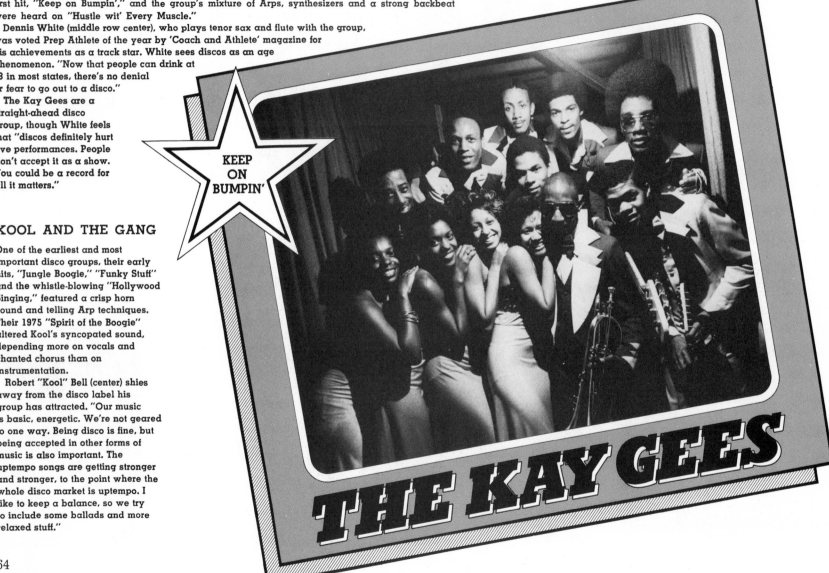

KEEP ON BUMPIN'

THE KAY GEES

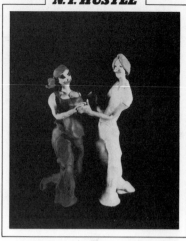

15) Gradually exaggerate this motion, until you are rocking while facing your clasped hands.

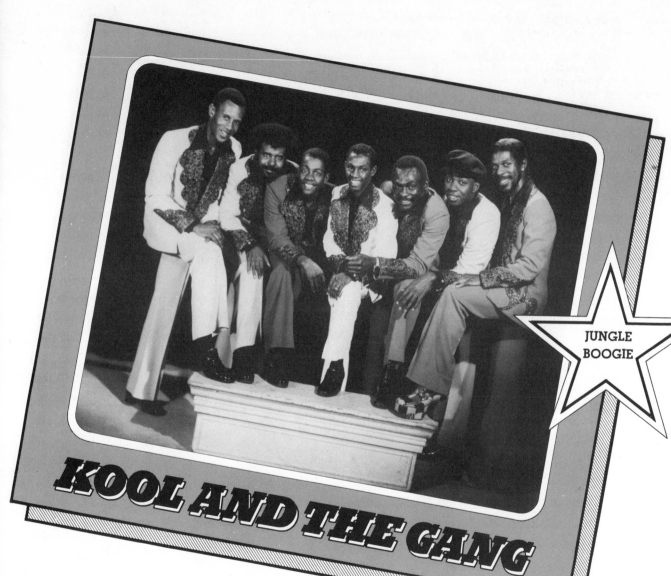

JUNGLE BOOGIE

KOOL AND THE GANG

2) Then swing your hips away from your partner, hopefully taking advantage of your natural sense of rhythm.

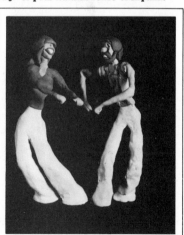

THE BUMP

TAVARES

Five brothers from Boston, Tavares developed a unique vocal blend as a ballad group with "She's Gone," then switched to uptempo disco. "It Only Takes a Minute," with close vocal harmonies over a strong rhythm track, certified their transition.

Their summer 1975 album, 'In the City,' which contained "Minute" and similar upbeat material, was a departure from their earlier style. "I think we'll be going disco for a while, until it stops," Butch Tavares (center) said. "Give people what they want. When they don't want it anymore, we'll start singing slow again."

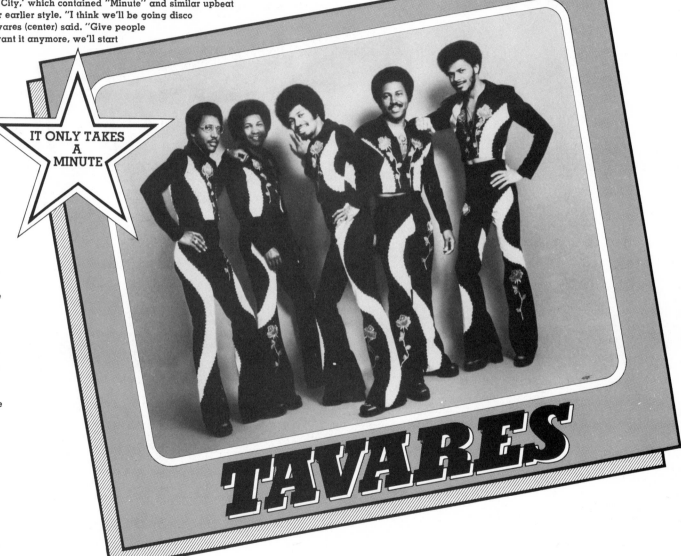

IT ONLY TAKES A MINUTE

TAVARES

DISCO-TEX

Aka Monti Rock III, Disco-Tex first came to America's attention as Johnny Carson's most frequent hair-dresser guest. His new incarnation as Disco-Tex came in 1974, when he entered the charts with the Bob Crewe/Kenny Nolan song, "Get Dancin'." "It took seven months of visiting every disco in America to break it," Tex shuddered. "It was the hardest job of my life. I've been dancing in discos for 12 years but never performed before this. It was a way of breaking a record, and the discotheque alone was the way I broke my record."

Disco-Tex's sound is bubblegum disco, relying on catchy lyrics rather than hot rhythms. But Disco-Tex doesn't seem concerned. "The disco craze is definitely a fad. I'm doing something brand-new next year."

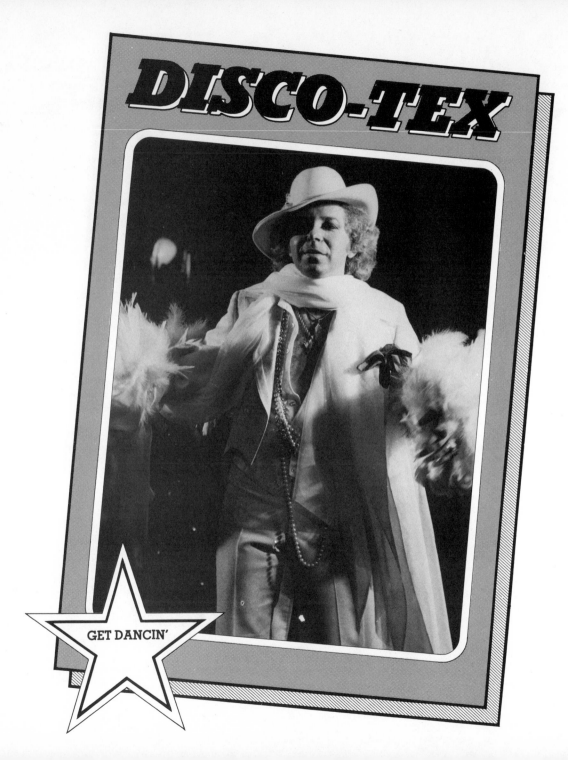

DISCO-TEX

GET DANCIN'

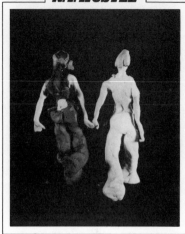

N.Y. HUSTLE

16) The man releases his right hand, the woman her left, and they turn outward until they are dancing side to side.

3) You can also bend your knees deeply and bump hips low.

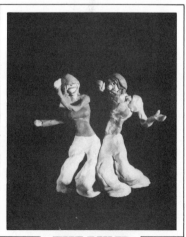

THE BUMP

PERCY FAITH

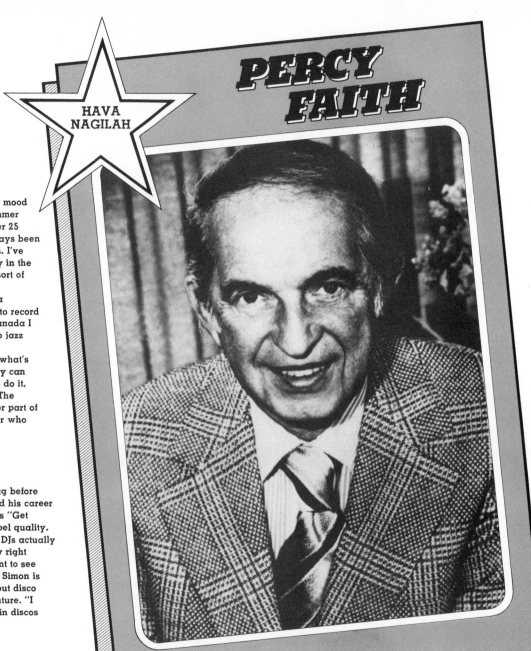

HAVA NAGILAH

PERCY FAITH

Well-known for his middle-of-the-road instrumental mood albums, the man who gave us "Theme from a Summer Place" has jumped on the disco bandwagon. "After 25 years with Columbia, I've run the gamut. I've always been in pop, and I ran out of new music after 80 albums. I've been studying contemporary music in order to stay in the business. Disco is the current trend, so my album sort of moved into discotheque mix."

'Disco Party,' Faith's "trendy" album, included a reworking of "Hava Nagilah." "I've had the idea to record 'Hava Nagilah' for years. When I was 23 up in Canada I played with a band where we'd put the classics to jazz and vice versa. It's a continuation of that."

Percy visits the discos occasionally "just to see what's going on." Of this album, he said, "Apparently they can dance to it. I don't have the physical equipment to do it, but as a musician I'm led into the right grooves." The album was designed so it wouldn't offend the older part of his audience. "I have to think in terms of the buyer who will get my record and dance at home."

JOE SIMON

Ballads and C&W-styled material were Simon's bag before "Get Down, Get Down (Get on the Floor)" propelled his career into the discos. Sung in a relaxed baritone, Simon's "Get Down" and "Music in My Bones" had a disco-gospel quality.

"Discos are exciting," Simon said, "because the DJs actually fight over records to break. They can let you know right away if you have a record and then we experiment to see if it's just for disco or also for the mass audience." Simon is thankful for his recent hits but has no illusions about disco being the wave of the future—or, at least, of his future. "I can't get too wrapped up in it. If you get hung up in discos and forget what you're doing, it hurts you."

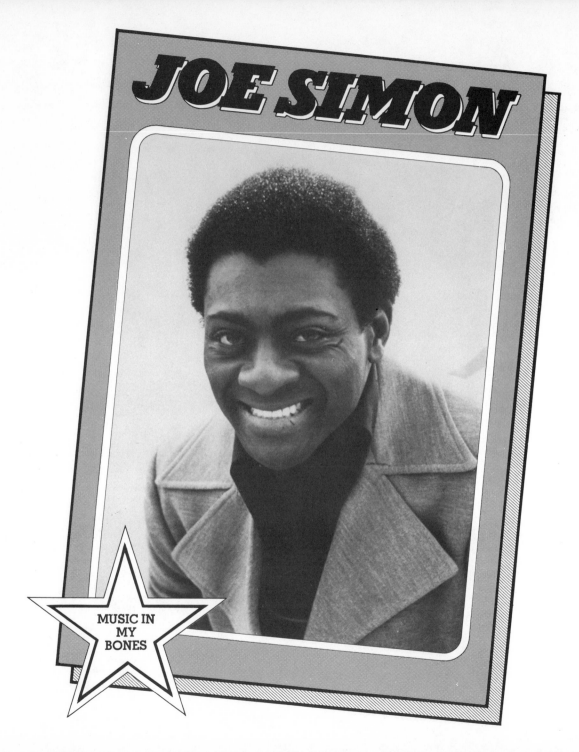

JOE SIMON

MUSIC IN MY BONES

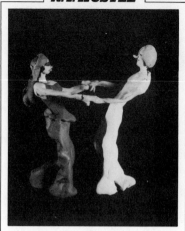

17) Try it a couple of times. Then take your partner's other hand, bop style, and stretch away from your partner before coming together with both hands still clasped. This pattern can be repeated until you're bored and ready to move on.

4) Vary hip bumping by bumping back to back, sticking your butt out behind you toward your partner and throwing your arms out in front of you. If you don't feel stupid doing this, then you're not doing it right.

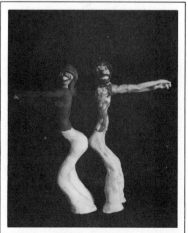

THE BUMP

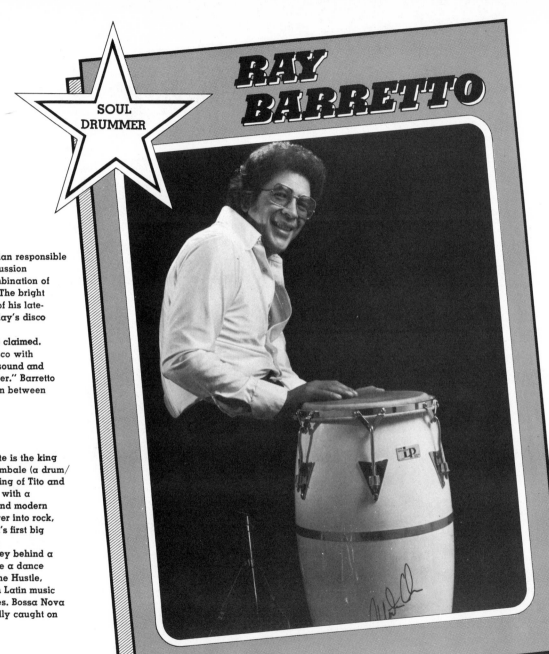

SOUL DRUMMER

RAY BARRETTO

RAY BARRETTO

Barretto is the bandleader and session musician responsible for establishing congas as a strong lead percussion instrument. Like Puente, Ray's music is a combination of musical styles, using Latin salsa as its base. The bright horn arrangements and conga syncopations of his late-Sixties "Soul Drummer" predated much of today's disco music.

"The sound in discos is the draw," Barretto claimed. "They can make a band sound better in a disco with their equipment. You're guaranteed that the sound and the atmosphere is going to be warm and sexier." Barretto predicted that "in the next year a combination between disco and salsa will be happening."

TITO PUENTE:

If James Brown is the godfather of soul, Puente is the king of Latin salsa music. For over 25 years, the timbale (a drum/cowbell combination played with sticks) playing of Tito and his orchestra has been filling Latin ballrooms with a distinctive sound that combines Afro-Cuban and modern pop/jazz influences. Tito has even crossed over into rock, writing the original version of one of Santana's first big hits, "Oye Como Va."

Tito believes that dance fads are the real key behind a music's success. "Any music that doesn't have a dance behind it won't make it. With the Bump and the Hustle, disco has dances to go with it. The same with Latin music and the Mambo, Samba and Merengue dances. Bossa Nova was a popular form of music, but it never really caught on because there was no dance to go with it."

TITO PUENTE

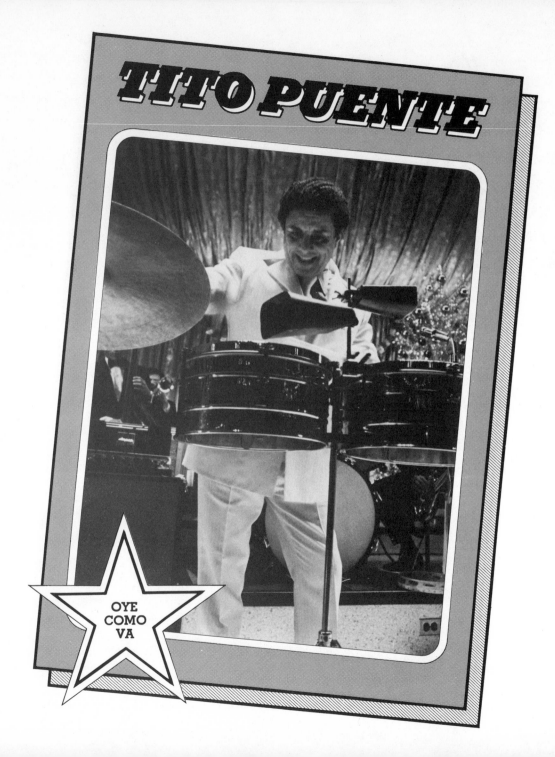

OYE COMO VA

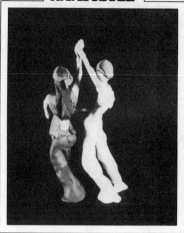

18) Now we'll do one wrap turn, a tricky step in which the woman should find herself leaning back against the man with her arms crossed straitjacket style. Starting with both hands clasped, the man raises his left arm across his body and . . .

5) You can bump shoulders . . .

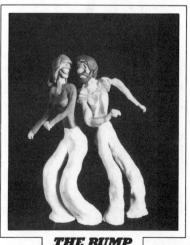

THE BUMP

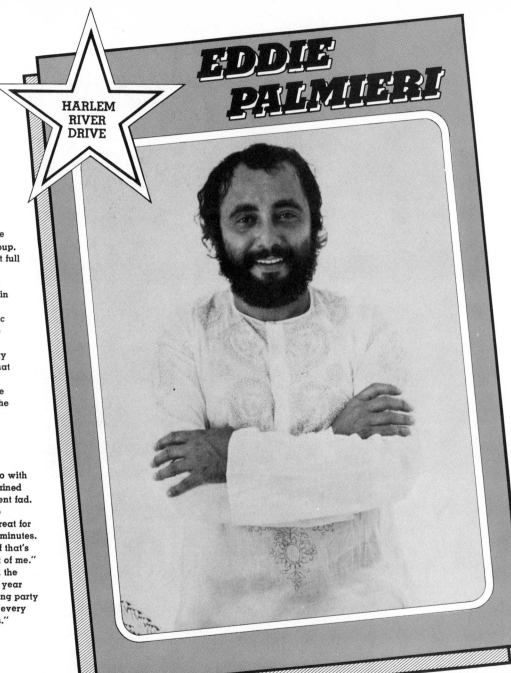

HARLEM RIVER DRIVE

EDDIE PALMIERI

EDDIE PALMIERI

The brash Palmieri plays keyboards in addition to producing and arranging his material. Eddie was responsible for recording one of the great Latin/soul fusion discs, "Harlem River Drive." Released in the late Sixties, when Santana was thought of as The Latin group. Palmieri's disc was New York tough, a pounding effort full of searing percussion and brilliant arrangements.

The disco crowd may prefer to dance rather than be entertained by a group, but the opposite is true for Latin dance freaks. "They'll come to where we're playing rather than go to the discos," Palmieri said. "Our music is unique and alive. Latins want to come and dance to a band, not a jukebox."

Eddie returned to New York in 1975 after a short stay in California. "The West Coast cannot comprehend what we're doing back here. They're out to lunch as far as Latin music goes. It's true they don't have the exposure to as many Latin bands, but that's because it's all in the East."

HERBIE MANN

A jazz flutist for some 20 years, Mann moved into disco with 1974-75's "Hijack." His followup LP, 'Waterbed,' contained less disco, reflecting Mann's displeasure with the current fad.

"Disco is like a great porno film," Mann said. "If the characters and filming technique are interesting, it's great for five minutes. That's what disco music is, good for five minutes. All the audience is interested in is tapping their feet. If that's all you want to hear, fantastic, but it bores the shit out of me."

Herbie has definite ideas about the disco image and the selling of it. He's visited a number of clubs in the past year but doesn't claim to have the clean-fun image of dancing party freaks. "Maybe I don't know the 'in' clubs to visit, but every disco I've been to is full of pimps, hookers and dealers."

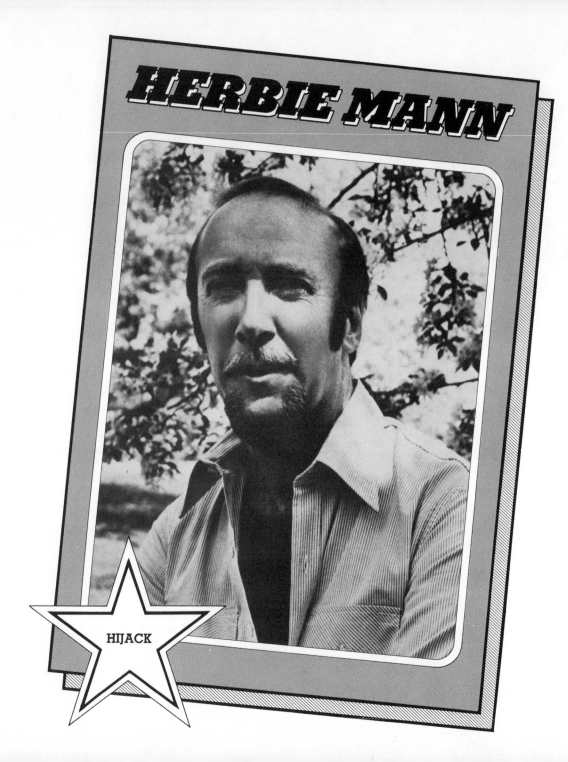

HERBIE MANN

HIJACK

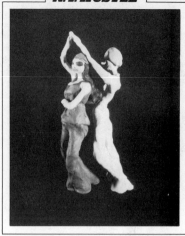

N.Y. HUSTLE

19) . . . turns the woman under it. If you both haven't let go, the woman now has her back to the man.

6) . . . or elbows . . .

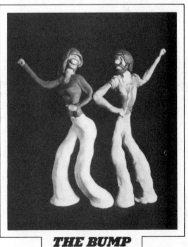

THE BUMP

BARRABAS

Barrabas is a six-man group from Spain that gained attention with the original version of "Hijack" which went on to win widespread disco play. "Our version of 'Hijack' was more popular than Herbie Mann's," lead singer José Luis (2nd from left) insisted. "We had more salsa."

The group itself is of mixed origin. The two guitarists, the Morales brothers, were born in Manila, while the keyboard artist comes from Portugal and the bass instrumentalist from Cuba. Only the drummer and Tejada are Spanish natives.

"It just happens that our mix of funk and Latin sounding rock & roll appeals to Americans," Morales mused. "We are already a success there. Atco sends us lists of discotheque successes with us at the top."

The guitarist admitted that "I don't go to discos in Spain. I don't go out in Madrid." Tejada said that "we get airplay in Madrid, but not as much as in New York City."

EARTH, WIND & FIRE

Led by Maurice White, who writes, produces and plays percussion, the group has perfected the Sly Stone sound heard on the energetic "Shining Star" and the more melodic, breezier "That's the Way of the World." Brassy arrangements. Aquarian-age lyrics and fine vocals meld together into a sound that has made the band possibly the world's most popular disco-related group. Known throughout the Orient, Africa and Europe, they have spent as much time on global tours as on Stateside circuits.

Why the global following? Drummer Ralph Johnson (2nd row right) said it's because their "music is earthy, danceable and covers all aspects relevant to the audience. It's got everything in it and it's not just something to sit and look at."

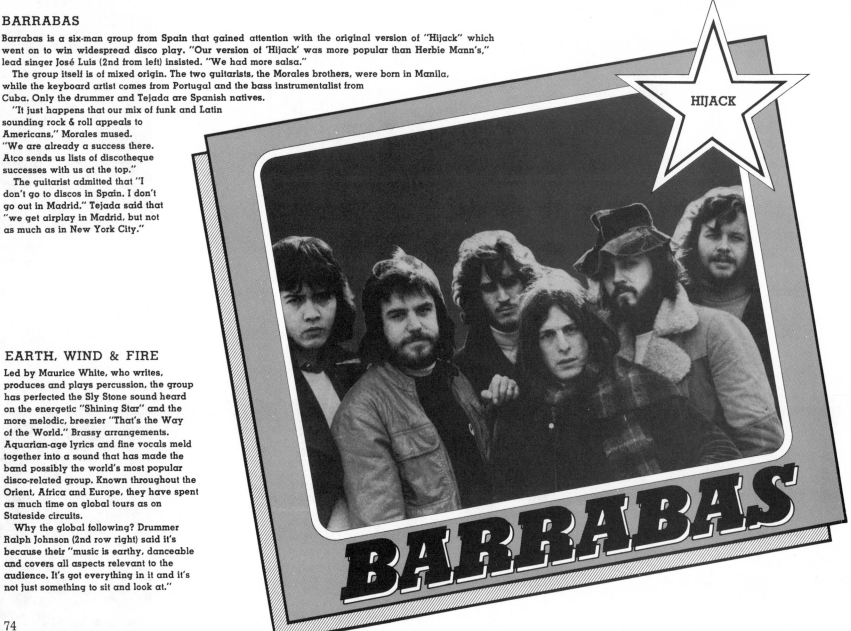

HIJACK

BARRABAS

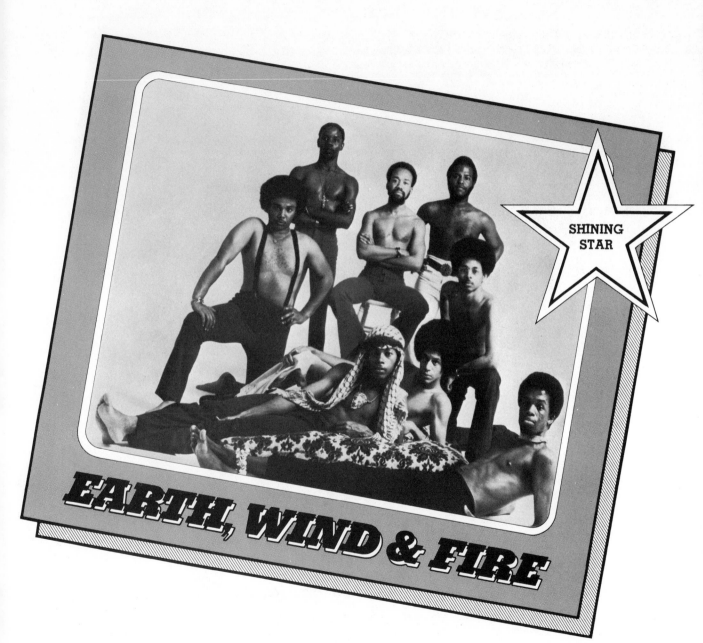

SHINING STAR

EARTH, WIND & FIRE

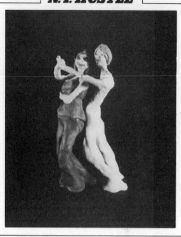

20) Now the man lowers his clasped hands in front of the woman . . .

7) . . . or knees—straight across . . .

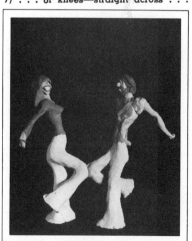

THE BUMP

SILVER CONVENTION

Originally consisting of three female backup singers, their first hit, "Save Me," was recorded as a one-take demo tape in a Munich studio. When the song clicked in Europe in spring 1975, a pickup touring band was added. Their producer, Michael Kunze, was a German folksinger and lyricist. "I planned them as a disco group," Kunze explained. "I don't go to discos very often, but when I went I realized all you needed was a strong bass line, a snappy snare sound and some coloring. You want to think, 'What will make the people dance.'"

"Save Me" originally broke the group in Europe, but it took "Fly, Robin, Fly" to bring international success. "All over the world there's an emerging disco culture," Kunze said. "It's an international culture following this brand of commercial soul music."

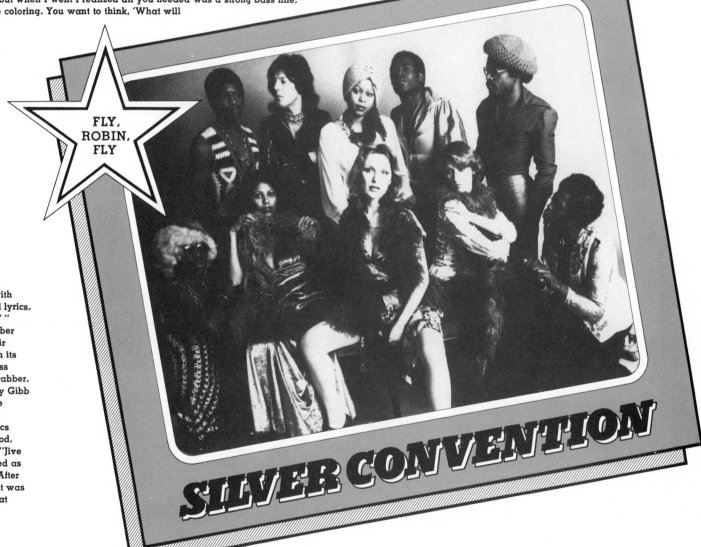

FLY, ROBIN, FLY

SILVER CONVENTION

BEE GEES

The three Gibb brothers have always done well in America with their vocal blend and thoughtful lyrics, but summer of '75's "Jive Talkin'" gave them a new brand of Number One song. A departure from their earlier lush style, "Talkin'," with its catchy refrain and dominant bass line, was an immediate disco grabber.

"People want to dance," Barry Gibb (lower right) said, explaining the change in the Bee Gees' music. "They're not listening to the lyrics anymore. They want to hear good, happy, stomp-your-feet music." "Jive Talkin'" was originally produced as an R&B single but, Gibb said, "After we recorded it everybody said it was disco. We didn't even know what disco was at the time."

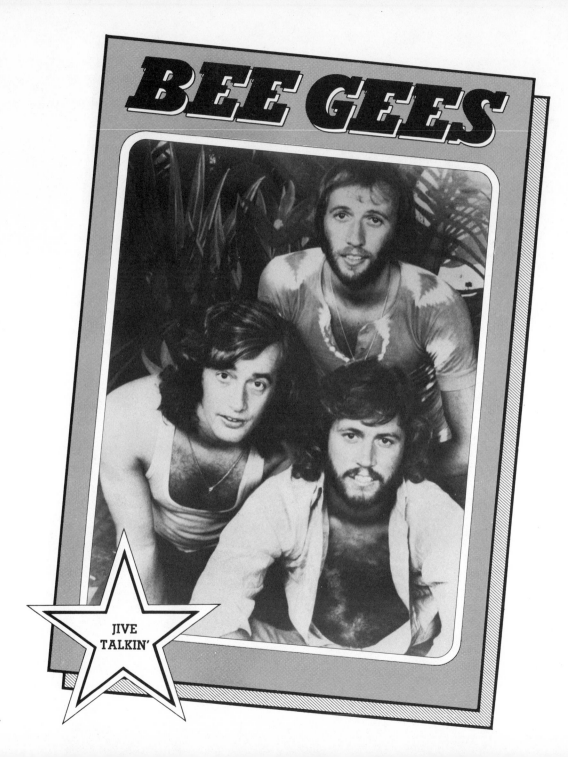

BEE GEES

JIVE TALKIN'

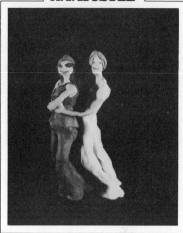

N.Y. HUSTLE

21) . . . so that her arms are crossed, his arm is around her and the two of you are still holding hands, rocking back and forth.

8) . . . or on a diagonal. Knees should be bumped (brushed might be safer) on the outside surface or even on the thigh rather than head-on. This may avoid painful accidents. When bumping your knees, throw your arms back for balance and effect.

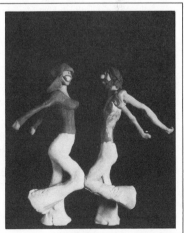

THE BUMP

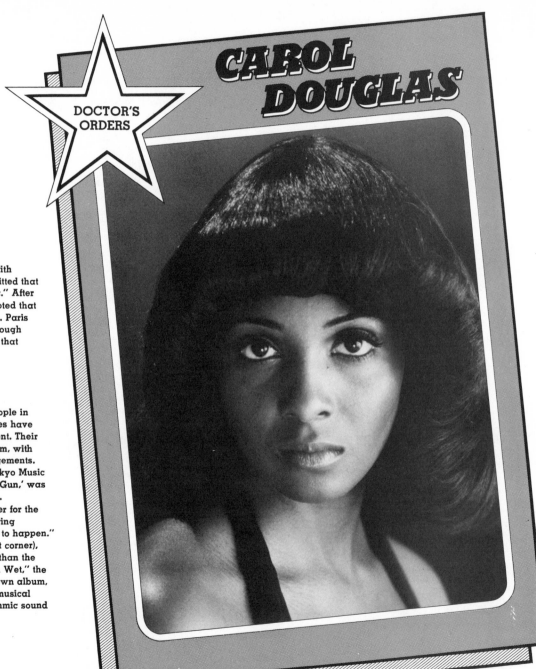

DOCTOR'S ORDERS

CAROL DOUGLAS

CAROL DOUGLAS

A former off-Broadway actress, Douglas scored with "Doctor's Orders" and "Headline News" but admitted that she'd "like to branch out into other types of music." After playing in discos on a 1975 European tour, she noted that "the disco scene over there is very similar to ours. Paris and Rome have discos much like New York's—though not as many. Everyone is doing the same dances that are popular here."

COMMODORES

Group trumpeter William King noted that "the people in the Orient are discotheque mad." The Commodores have capitalized on this madness with tours of the Orient. Their last two tours to the Philippines amazed even them, with 130,000 sold-out seats during both four-day engagements. They also won best singers award at the 1975 Tokyo Music Festival, and their first Motown album, 'Machine Gun,' was the largest-selling record in the history of Nigeria.

Walter Orange (top row, 2nd from left), drummer for the group, attributed their global success to their touring at a time when "the disco thing was first starting to happen." According to guitarist Tommy McClary (upper left corner), "A lot of countries seemed to be onto disco more than the States." But McClary, who wrote "Slippery When Wet," the Stevie Wonder-ish hit heard on their second Motown album, 'Caught in the Act,' added, "America is still the musical trendsetter in the world. With our energetic, rhythmic sound we gave them something to hang their hats on."

78

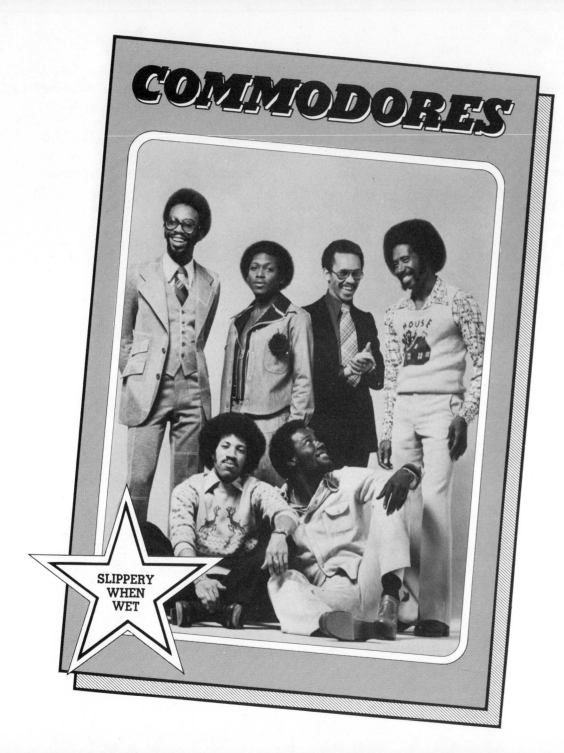

COMMODORES

SLIPPERY
WHEN
WET

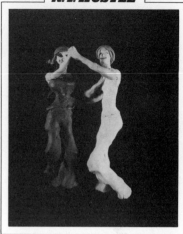

N.Y. HUSTLE

22) If you got into this, you can bloody well get yourselves out of it and back into a somewhat normal position . . . after which you'll be content to resume the Social Dance Position and talk about baseball.

9) If you want to surprise your partner, swing around on the off beat and bump his or her hips with your shoulder. Try turning around a lot, bumping with whatever's handy when you complete the circle.

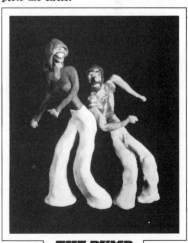

THE BUMP

FRANCE

France is where the disco originated, evolving from the Parisian tango club of the Twenties through the live-jazz "whiskey club" of the Fifties into the recorded-music bars of the last two decades. Still, most of the music played in Paris's 150 or so discos tends to be imported; "The Hustle," Esther Phillips's "What a Difference a Day Makes" and "I'm on Fire" (the British cut by 5000 Volts, not the Dwight Twilley Band's U.S. country rocker) were the Big Songs for '75. Barry White is out, the Philly sound and African-influenced music are on the rise.

Clubs like the Bus Palladium, the Whiskey A Go-Go and the Scottish Club start late and end much later. Admissions run in the 25-30 franc ($6-7) range, but many places toss in a free drink to soften the tariff. Disco radio is weak, centering around summertime shows broadcast from the various discos.

South on the Riviera, Les Frères de la Côte (the Brothers of the Coast), on the beach at Menton, hosts a youngish crowd that dances to French rock, reggae and an occasional Cha-Cha. In neighboring Monaco, jet-setters young and old take some Sinatra with their soul music at the swank New Jimmy's, dancing on a shiny sublit electric dance floor.

ENGLAND

The English disco scene which exploded along with Beatlemania got its second wind around 1970. There are now an estimated 30,000 disco parties going on in England on any Saturday night. British DJs have become virtual pop stars, with fan clubs and, occasionally, recording contracts. The British musicians' union feels threatened by the discos, especially the mobile shows which, complete with trucks, roadies, equipment and a library of as many as 500 singles and 100 LPs, hire out like a band to play at pubs, weddings, parties and even corporation dinners.

Typical is the Tom Cat Show, run by DJ Don Wilby, who carries with him 11,000 watts' worth of amplification, several decks, strobe lights, projectors and even gun powder flashes all packed into two trucks. Wilby, age 24, started out to become a singer, but the economics of the situation persuaded him to become a mobile DJ. "Why pay 50 pounds for a band," Wilby told *Melody Maker* magazine, "when you can pay 12 pounds for a disco?"

English dancers have taken to the disco shows not only because they are cheaper than live concerts, but because the action is nonstop. In order to work at all in England, some bands have had to turn themselves into human disco shows, cranking out nonstop re-creations of current hits. But as far as DJs like Wilby are concerned, the bands are doing it the hard way. "We're just like a pop group," Wilby continued, describing his show. "We have our own signature tune and a backup jock who plays slow records before I come on. There is a burst of machine-gun fire and then I hit the stage, the strobes come on, and for the next two hours it's write home and tell your mother."

Reggae is especially popular, as is a phenomenon known as "Northern Soul," which created a demand for obscure U.S. soul and R&B singles.

DISCO 'ROUND THE WORLD

Dancing to the Beat of the Global Village
Compiled by Frank Robertson

Thanks and a tip of the disco hat to Joe Cunningham, Jay Grossman, Paul Gambaccini and Melody Maker magazine, with special thanks to Billboard Publications.

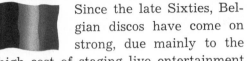

BELGIUM

Since the late Sixties, Belgian discos have come on strong, due mainly to the high cost of staging live entertainment and the availability of sophisticated record-playing hardware. Most clubs are open until 2:00 a.m., cater to teenagers and play established soul music and rock hits. Many discotheques are set in the huge Belgian roadside cafes, which can entertain and feed a crowd of 500. The roadside discos appeal to an older crowd —50-year-olds—and play old-time dance records.

Record companies do not promote their products through discos as they do in New York or England. Nevertheless, U.S. disco stars like Barry White and Shirley & Co. are big in Belgium where they've toured the country with live shows.

ITALY

Since 1972 Italian discotheques have multiplied to become practically the only game in town for Italian rock fans. The reason: A passion for music and a shaky national economy caused rioting at pop concerts and demands for free entertainment. The result: No concerts, not even free ones, because they're too risky for both promoters and performers. "Try to hold a free concert by the Rolling Stones here," one Italian promoter told *Billboard* magazine, "and 250,000 people who can't get in will show up and level the place."

Italian ballroom managers have discovered that it's safer—and cheaper—to hire a one-man band—the DJ—instead of a group. Italian discos, numbering over 1000, play international soul music, jazz, rock and Italian hits, a few of them serving as "test pilots" for up-and-coming live talent.

WEST GERMANY

In West Germany there is a disco to satisfy even the most jaded palate. Want Lou Reed's music and a decadently postured clientele? Try Tiffany's in Munich. Barry White-Philly sound? Walk into any big-city disco. Low-volume MOR? You'll find that too.

The first West German disco opened in 1959; today there are approximately 3500—all thriving as German record consumers devour the disco sound. James Last's *Non-Stop Dancing 20* sold 250,000 copies in one month, and Ariola-Eurodisc has put out a series of classical music LPs—from Bach to Ravel—optimistically titled *Discotheque of the Masters*. West German disco DJs are relatively well-paid ($800 a month) and are regarded as intellectuals.

CANADA

 The "World's Biggest Disco Party" was thrown by a Canadian/U.S. promotion team during June 1975 in the Montreal Forum. Over 7000 people showed up for nearly five hours of nonstop dancing, with disco DJs playing records between live performances by Van McCoy (whose "Disco Baby" sold 15,000 copies in the Montreal area the day it was released), Gloria Gaynor and Shirley & Co.

Discos in Quebec have become reliable indexes of coming hit soul singles, and record companies watch such places as Dominique's, the Speakeasy, Lime Light, Harlow's, Valentino and the 2001 Coupes in Montreal for dollar signs. West coast Canada is more of a disco frontier. In British Columbia the citizenry only recently decreed it legal to dance in many of the region's restaurants and "beer parlors." Sgt. Pepper's, a disco franchise chain, is planning to leap into the breach in Calgary and Winnipeg.

MEXICO

 Mexico's disco action is concentrated in resort areas such as Acapulco, where Mexican and U.S. tourists may dance to five or six in the morning. The music is loud American R&B featuring lots of Barry White, with the creative Mexican DJs integrating sound effects—a jet taking off, a train passing—into the music. Bill Haley and Chubby Checker are still played, and although they love to Bump, Mexican disco dancers would just as soon do the Twist, the Cancan, the Mexican Hat Dance or the Jitterbug to "Rock Around the Clock."

SPAIN

 There are 9000 discotheques in dance-crazy Spain. They're open from six in the evening to ten, when they close for a while so everyone can rest, eat, primp and regroup. The discos reopen about eleven and go until four in the morning. The DJs like to radically change the style of music every half-hour or so; a Spanish DJ may start out with some soul music, switch to bubblegum, then spin Spanish or American MOR, followed by traditional flamenco.

NETHERLANDS

 Although Dutch record companies don't see discos as important promotional outlets, there are many clubs in major cities. They offer a low-key atmosphere more conducive to conversation than dancing, and a token DJ plays popular requests and soul music. Most Dutch discos consider themselves membership-only clubs, but they will admit anyone who looks "reasonable." The most innovative disco form in the Netherlands is a drive-in show featuring popular radio DJs who visit rural areas.

An increase in the price of singles has prompted a Dutch consumer-action group, Singles Boycott 1975-1978, to threaten action against any price hikes on Dutch singles. In 1975 a single sold for—ready? —$2.45.

RUSSIA

 No one would ever suggest that the Russians, who gave us vodka and the Bolshoi, aren't into music and dancing. But discos . . . well, remember, it's the Soviet Union and as recently as 1973 the Russians were still making 78s. They do have jukeboxes there, but they're programmed with Brenda Lee, Englebert Humperdinck and Andy Williams records—although occasionally you do find some Stones and Beatles tunes.

Russians do buy a lot of records to play on predominantly mono hi-fis, but it's still news in Russia when the Leningrad Dixieland Band has to cancel gigs because the clarinetist is sick.

POLAND

 Discos are becoming popular in Poland, playing American and Western European records, plus some Hungarian hits. Polish DJs have all been organized in one trade union—under government control, of course—and aspiring new DJs are "examined" by a special commission nominated by the Ministry of Culture and Art. Applicants are expected to have a respectable knowledge of music and a high-school diploma.

Although there is a great demand for them, singles have been almost non-existent on the Polish market. The country's only record company, Polskie Nagrania, is just beginning to release them for discotheque presentation; title selection is in the hands of another special commission. Records made for the discos can be bought only in discos, not in record stores.

DENMARK

 Denmark's largest chain of discos, Torkenskiold (named for a Danish war hero), offers lavish interiors—silk, carpets, antiques—as well as occasional live entertainment.

The record companies have paid close attention to the disco scene since George McCrae's "Rock Your Baby" broke there. But the latest thing in Denmark is the videotheque, where you may see and hear an artist performing on videotape while you dance.

FINLAND

There is a quietly thriving disco scene in Finland, with about 300 permanent clubs (plus traveling discos). The best-known DJs enjoy a following similar to that of Top 20 pop singers. About half the clubs sell booze, hence teenagers are not allowed in—there are only two clubs for them in Helsinki, the Luola and the Catacombi. International soul music is favored along with rockers like Gary Glitter, Suzi Quatro, Mud, Nazareth and Alvin Stardust. The more mature discogoers, and there are a lot of them in Finland, prefer traditional rock from Bill Haley, Elvis and Paul Anka, soul music and the Philadelphia sound. Music volume in Finland's discos is limited by law to 85 decibels, and expensive apparatus has been installed in some clubs for measuring loudness. Finnish DJs wear protective headphones and they complain that it is hard to get people dancing at only 85 decibels.

AUSTRALIA

The disco scene is starting to boom in Australia. In Sydney, the Hyatt Kingsgate's Mayfair nightclub was doing poorly until it changed its name to Trinkets, went disco and began to attract a couple thousand people a week.

JAPAN

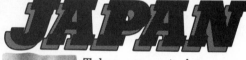

Tokyo seems to have more discos than any city in the world, although to the Japanese "disco" means any place that serves up a disco sound, be it a live band, recorded music or both. Some "discos" are coffeehouses with a good sound system but no dance floor—just students drinking strong coffee and listening to 100 decibel music. Japan follows the U.S. hit parade and keeps a close watch on the U.S. music scene via the Armed Forces Network, on which you can hear Wolfman Jack five nights a week.

Tokyo's "disco shrine" is the Mugen-Byblos combination—two clubs under one management located next door to one another. Mugen ("eternity") is mainly a live-music saloon specializing in funk—they have house soul bands imported from the States—and occasional big-name acts like Ike and Tina Turner, the Three Degrees and the Pointer Sisters. When the band breaks at Mugen, a DJ booth on a boom descends over the dance floor to blast 350 watts of sound through the JBL PA speakers. Mugen closes at 12:30, but next door Byblos is just getting started and doesn't stop until 4:00 a.m. The Hardcore pass between Byblos's twin seven-foot statues of Athena and dance in a multileveled cavelike atmosphere while the DJ rides from level to level in his mobile booth.

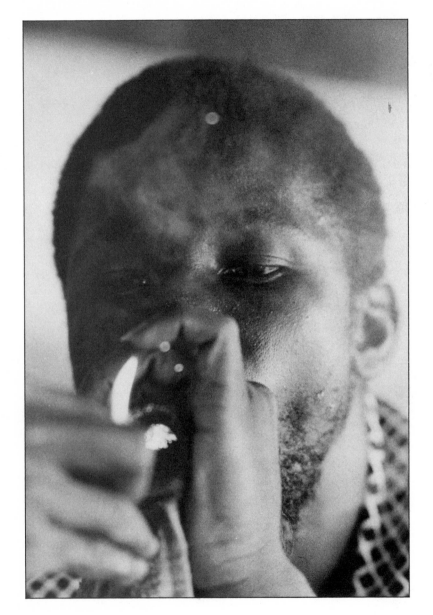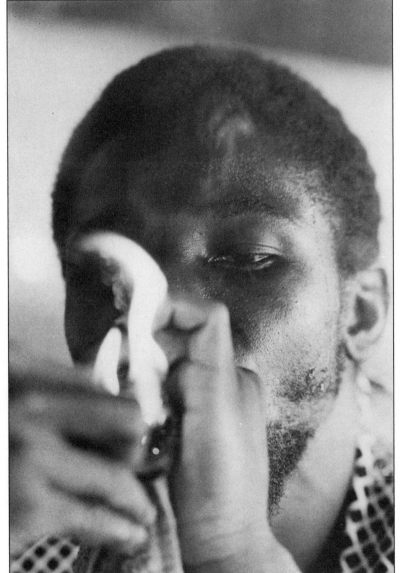

'HI, I'M TOOTS HIBBERT

and I'm Going to Teach You to Dance to Reggae'

When we play in Jamaica, everybody is up dancin'—nobody just sit and watch. Reggae came out of nowhere; it's just from sufferation and poverty. You have to suffer to know how to do it. It sounds so simple, yet it's so hard to play.

"In reggae, the beat came before the dance. The idea of the beat is you have the drum casting around, playing off the beat. The bass line goes with it. The rhythm guitar strides right on through—one, two, three, four.

"When you dance, you dance right on the beat. It's a feeling—if you can't feel the beat, you can't do the dance. You dance it however you want to dance—with your feet or with

---

Vocalist and composer Frederick Hibbert, the "Toots" of Toots and the Maytals, is the originator of the term "reggae" and perhaps the most popular artist in Jamaica today.

your hands. The key is: Follow the bass. The drum beat will lure you, but straddle it and the bass will carry you along.

"Reggae came from the ska beat. The ska beat was the fastest. Then the rock steady beat was a little slower. To do rock steady you just stay in one place and rock it. Reggae's like the rock steady beat, but it's a little slower and heavier.

"In reggae you have different moves, different dances. The Suzuki you dance on the palms of your feet; your feet move like a broom sweeping 'round and 'round. The Ride-a-Bike is another one. The Ride-a-Bike is just the way you sit on a bike. Knees in, toes out, holding the handlebars. You shake up and down, and turn about like you're riding into a deep corner. The Chuckie is popular; it's the one you hear more about. The Chuckie is a revolution dance; when you do the Chuckie you have to have a towel in your back pocket to dry off your face."

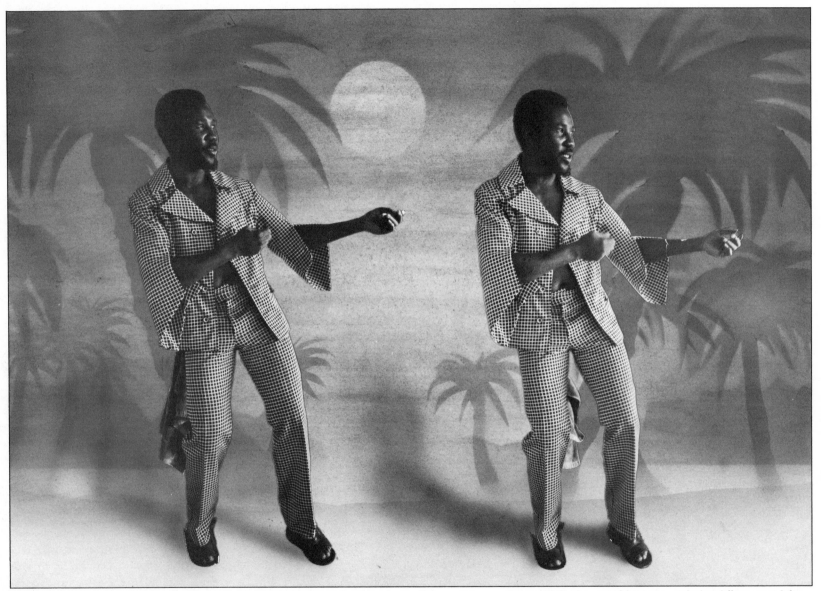

CHUCKIE 1) Move your left foot to the side on the first beat, move your hands and arms the way you are going . . . 2) On the second beat your right foot follows your left.

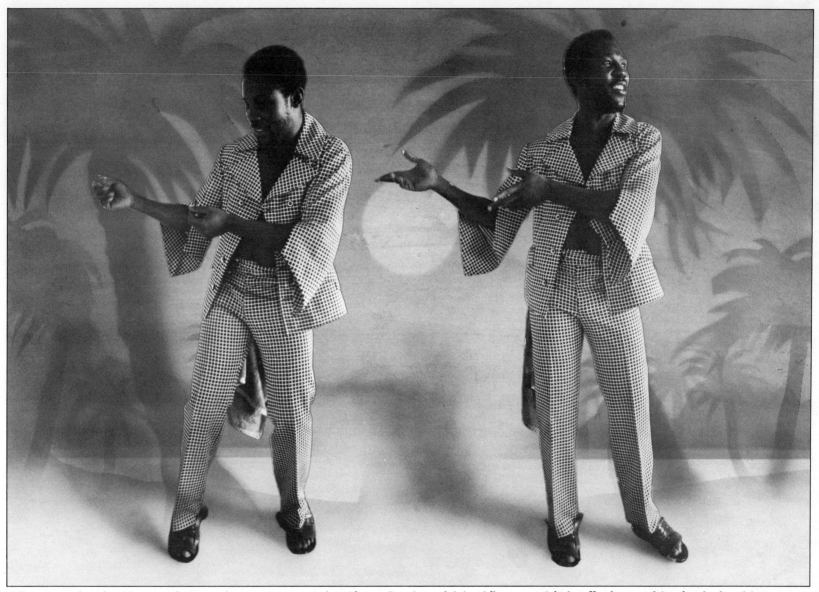

3) Then step to the side with your right foot, and move your arms to that side . . . 4) and your left foot follows your right foot. You keep on doing that, back and forth.

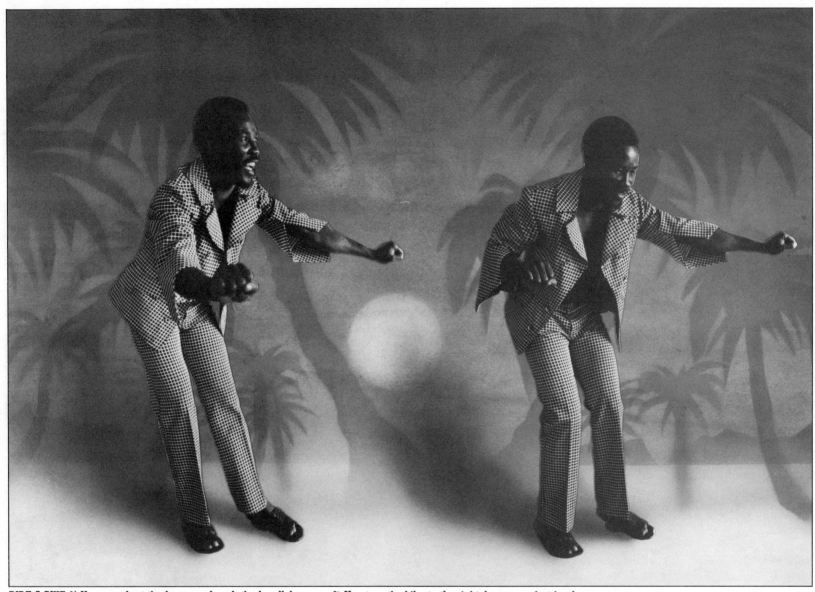

RIDE-A-BIKE 1) You crouch at the knees and grab the handlebars . . . 2) You turn the bike to the right, keep your feet in place.

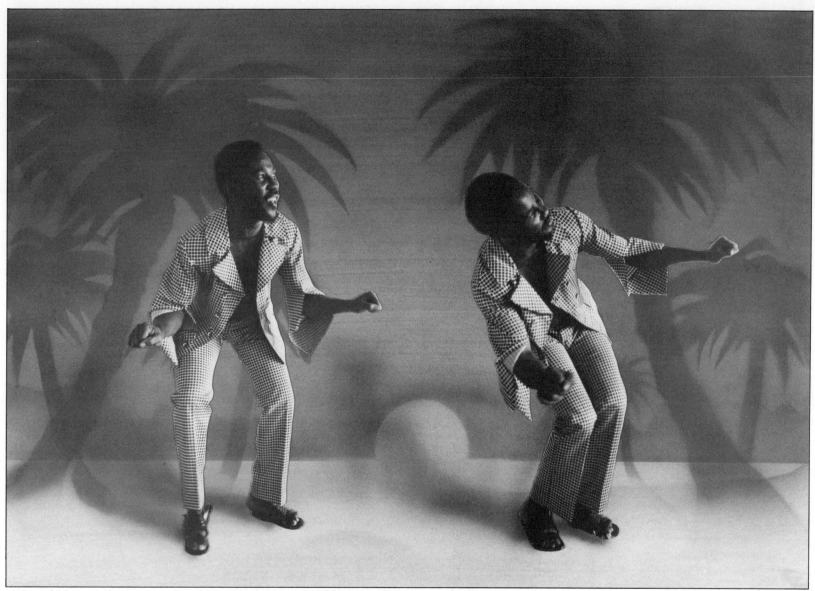

3) Get right down on that curve . . . 4) and swivel back to the left and keep on ridin'.

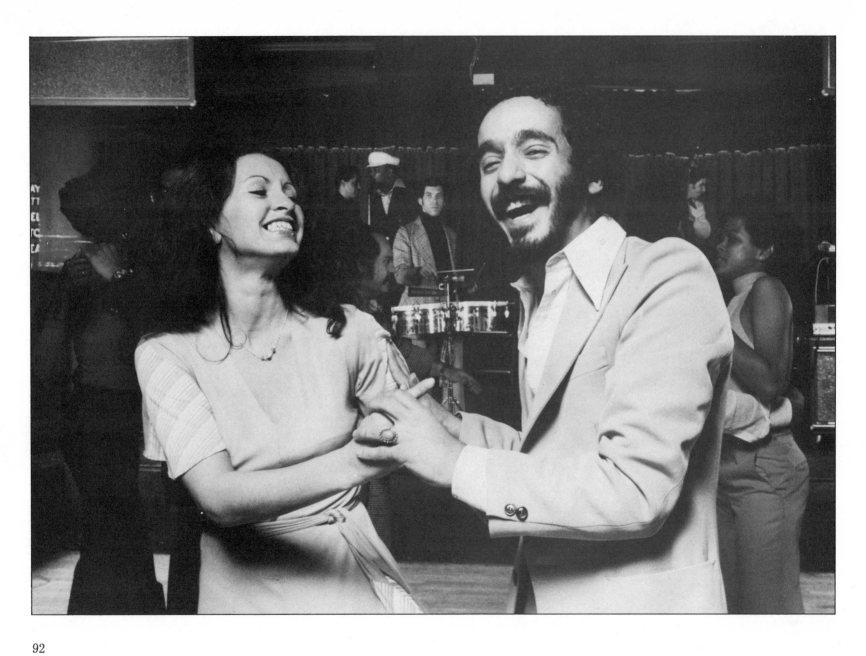

"HI, I'M WILLIE COLON

and I'm Going to Teach You to Dance to Salsa'

ey, there—*Que pasa?* I'm Willie Colon, and I'm with Iris Feliciano at The Corso club in New York, where my friend Ernie Agosto's La Conspiracion is playing, to show you how to dance to the New York Latin sound we call salsa. I think you'll dig doing it, and it'll help you get into the music too, because dancing is what salsa's all about. Why, even Eddie Palmieri calls his band 'the orchestra of the happy feet,' and Eddie's into some heavy head music!

"The basic steps are the same for all the different rhythms of salsa, and the basic beat is always four-quarter time—four

Willie Colon, 25-year-old bandleader, composer and trombonist, came out of the South Bronx at age 17 to build a constituency that extends from his neighborhood to Central America.

beats to the measure. That's important because you move your feet on three of these beats, the second, third and fourth, and you hold on the first. If you try to dance on the first beat you'll be fighting the whole flow of the rhythm.

"Secondly, take it easy! Most everything today is uptempo, is salsa, but you can't expect to get out there and dance uptempo straightaway. You have to associate each step with the proper beat, and if you try to do that to a fast rhythm, you'll be in trouble. So start with something slow—even a cha-cha-cha—and gradually up the tempo until you can dance at any speed and be cool.

"I'm going to give you the man's steps, but the man and the woman alternate patterns. That's to say, when he's coming forward on his left, she's going back on her right and so on. Okay so far? *Chévere*, let's do it."

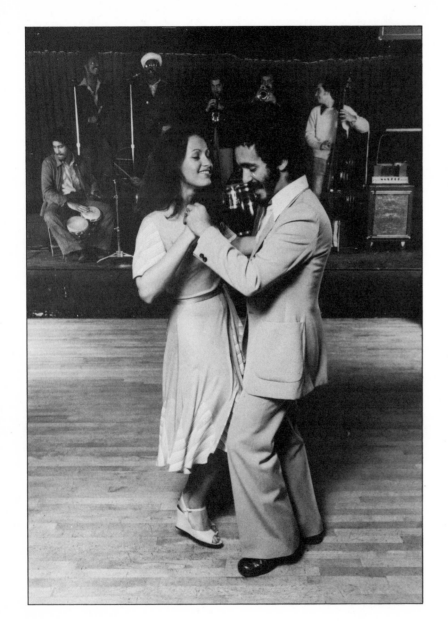

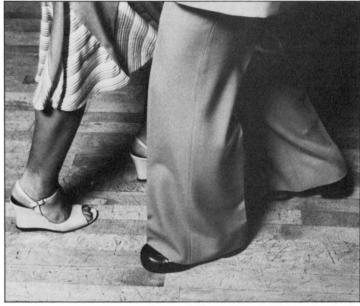

1) (pictured at left) On the first beat I do nothing—I'm just ready to start.
2) (above) On the second beat of the measure
my first step is forward on my left foot.

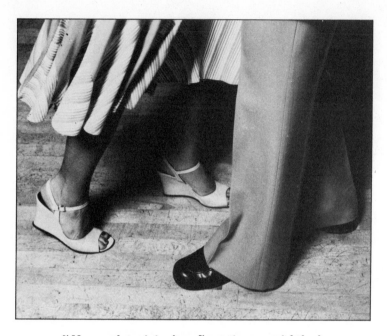

3) My second step is in place; I'm putting my weight back onto my right foot without moving either foot.

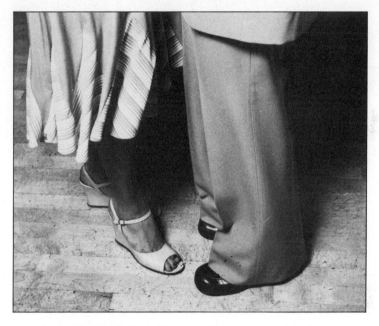

4) (above) For my third step, I'm moving my left foot backward so my feet are together on the last beat of the measure. It's a passing step, so my left foot actually comes down just slightly behind my right.

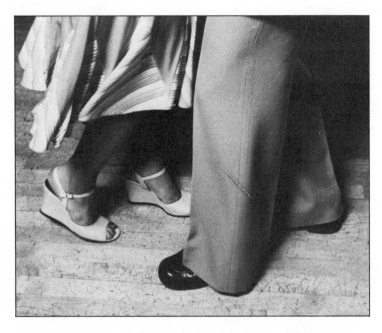 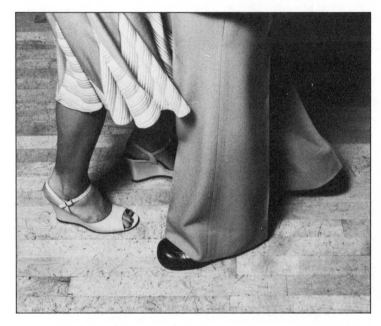

5) (not shown) Now I hold for the first beat of the next measure. My feet don't move, though my body still moves back slightly because this is a flowing movement. 6) (above) On the second beat I step back onto the ball of my right foot. All the other steps are onto the flat of my foot, but that'd make this back step jerky.

7) (above) On the third beat I step in place on my left foot, shifting my weight forward a little. 8) (pictured at right) Lastly, I bring my feet almost together again by moving my right foot forward.

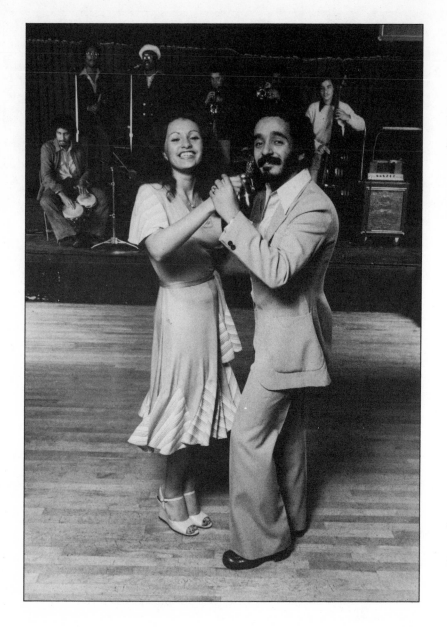

SOME SALSA TIPS: The basic pattern has six steps, spread over eight beats. You never take two consecutive steps on the same foot and your weight always goes to the foot you're stepping on.

"The whole thing has to flow. Even on the holding beat, your body keeps moving in the direction you'll be going on the next step.

"You'll always start together, in the ballroom hold, and move 'round slowly to the man's left as you dance. Your variations can happen on any of the beats, but you should always be dancing within that basic rhythm pattern. That means you can come back to your partner without any hesitation and stumbling, with the man still going forward on his left foot, and the woman going back on her right.

"There's a release where you break away and do what we call open work. The open work itself is mostly about body movement and any steps you need to get there. A lot of time there will be turns where the woman spins under the man's left arm, for example, and back again, and then maybe he'll go a turn under hers. Then you also break away completely and improvise face to face.

"The hand movements flow naturally from the body movements; no fancy gyrations or wild stuff. Keep them up around chest height. Basically, it's anything that's comfortable and doesn't look grotesque.

"One last thing. Don't talk about 'dancing the salsa.' Salsa is the music. You don't talk about 'dancing the rock,' do you?"—W.C.

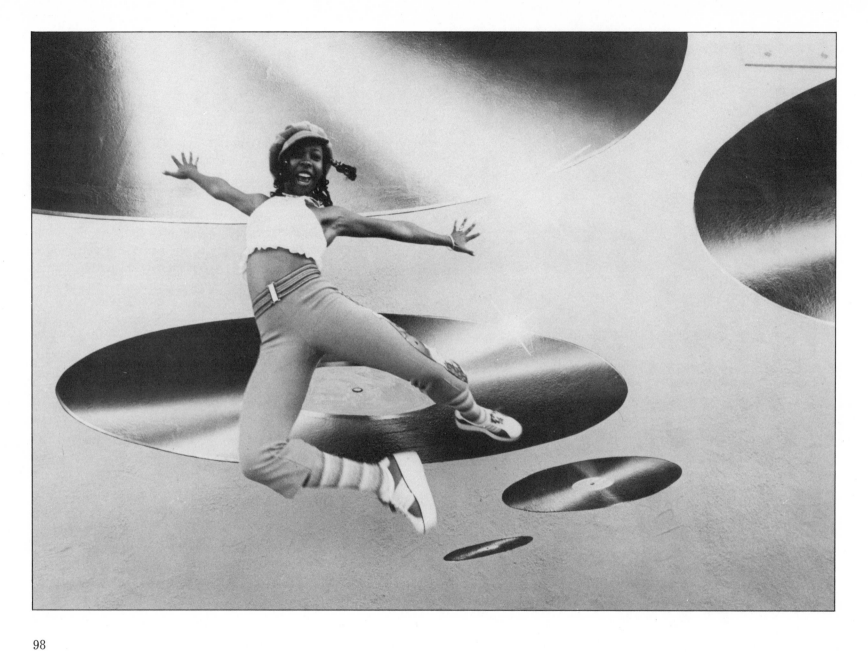

"HI, I'M DAMITA JO FREEMAN

and I'm Going to Teach You to Dance Funky like on 'Soul Train'

Here are three dances I helped make up which have caught on with the other kids in the *Soul Train* gang. When I went to Los Angeles's Crenshaw High, the girls there called me 'Rubberlegs' —but just 'cause you can't kick as high or bend as low shouldn't scare you off. These dances should reflect your personality and your imagination. They should become *your* dances.

"In almost all my dances I step back with the leg that is on the opposite side of the arm that is thrusting forward. I guess I'm just an opposite kid. Actually, when you walk, you walk opposite—your right leg goes forward and your left arm goes up. Since dancing should feel as natural as walking, mostly every dance here is an opposite arm/opposite leg dance.

"One of the most popular dances to come out of *Soul Train* is the Lock, which I learned from Don Campbell. The Lock is basically a hip-and-knee dance, so always remember to bend the knee and then straighten it out.

"The Breakdown is a dance I like 'cause you don't move your feet at all. In this variation, the only movement is in your hips, knees and arms and, of course, your head. If you do it in slow motion you can break down the steps and see how your hips, legs and head move.

"The Scooby Doo is a jump-kick dance which is frantic and which I guarantee will get you noticed at any party you go to.

"Once you have those three movements mastered you have most of the dances we do."

'Soul Train' went on television in 1971. The next year Damita Jo Freeman, currently a regular on the show, won a dance contest in her first appearance. Her partner was Don Campbell, who later went on to form the Lockers.

THE LOCK STEP

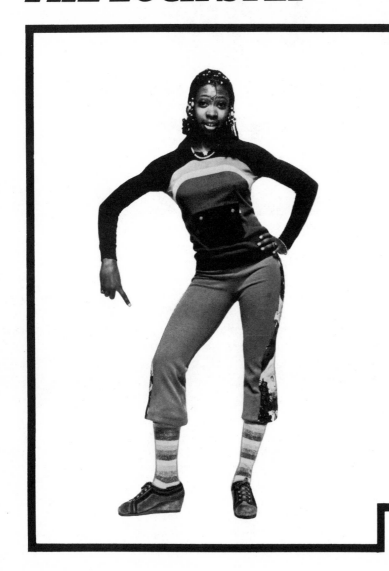

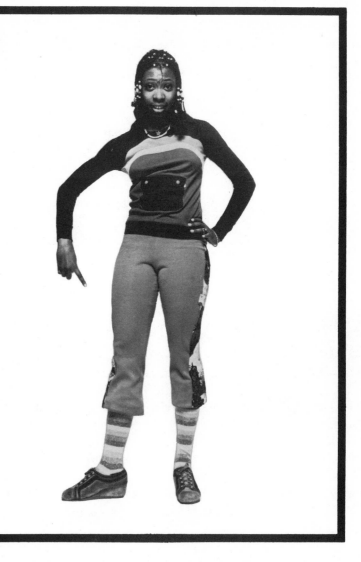

The Lock is basically a hip and knee movement, so always remember to bend your knee . . . and then straighten it out.

100

THE BASIC LOCK

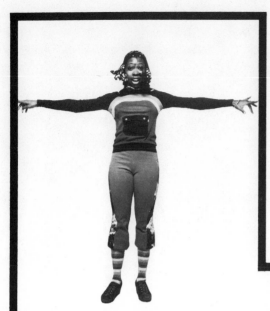

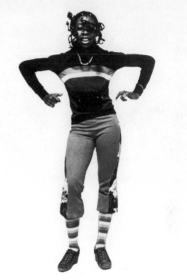

Now you're ready for the Basic Lock: (counterclockwise) 1) Stretch out your arms with your right leg a little in front of your left. 2) Throw your hands up and look to the sky. 3) Bend your knee and point your elbows skyward. 4) Do another Lock, but jiggle your hip from the left to the right and move your knees back and forth.

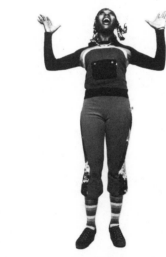

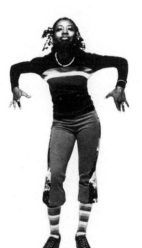

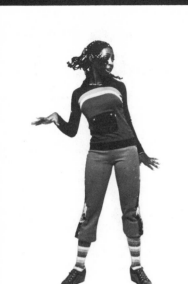

THE BREAK-DOWN

The Breakdown (counterclockwise): 1) You rock to the side, let's say the left, with your knees straight. 2) Now you swing your right hip out and throw your right arm behind you. 3) Use your head to make the style. 4) The arm that goes behind you should be on the same side of your body as the hip that is being moved to the side.

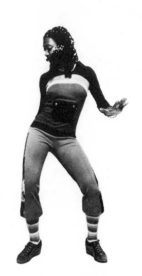

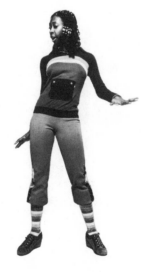

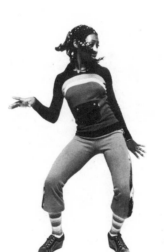

THE SCOOBY DOO

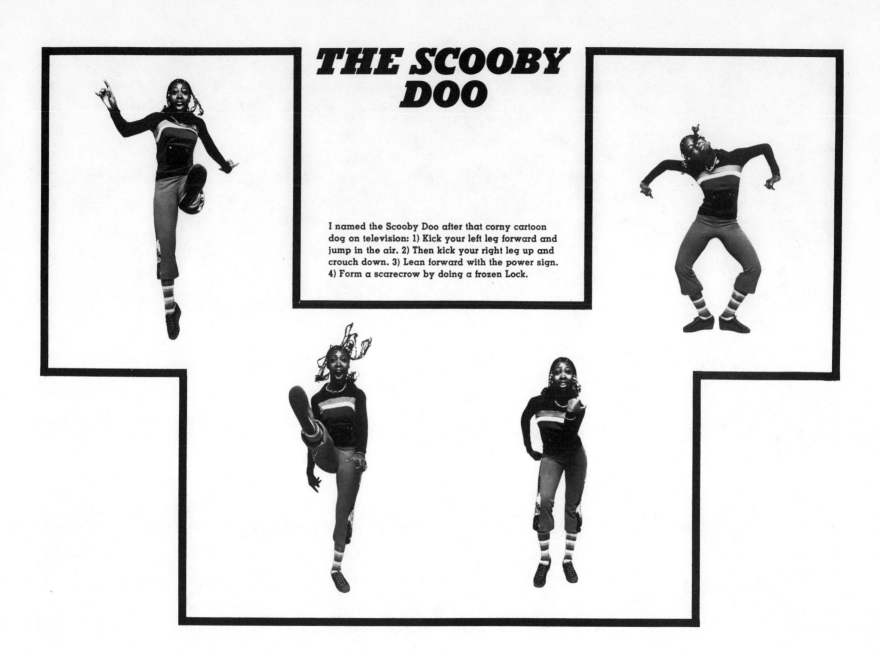

I named the Scooby Doo after that corny cartoon dog on television: 1) Kick your left leg forward and jump in the air. 2) Then kick your right leg up and crouch down. 3) Lean forward with the power sign. 4) Form a scarecrow by doing a frozen Lock.

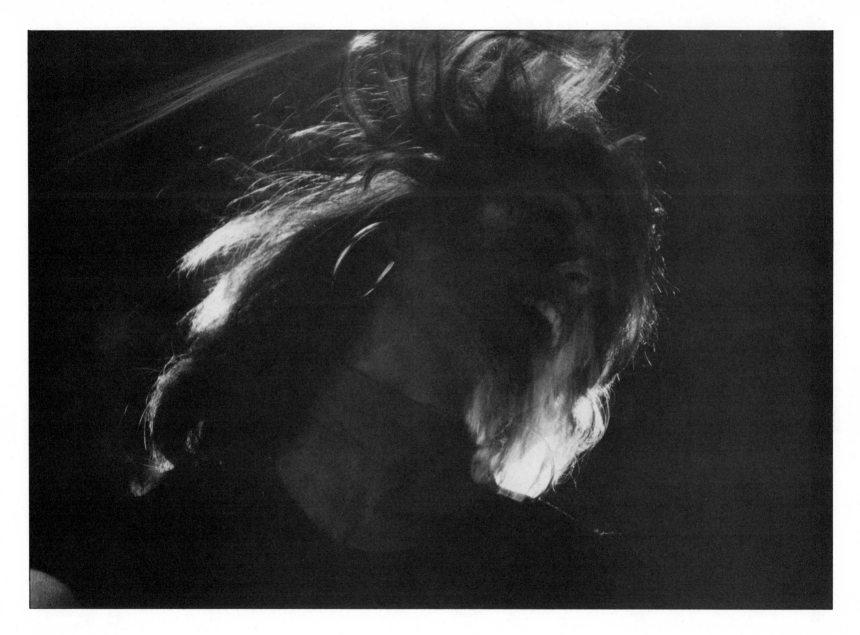

'Hi, I'm Karen Lustgarten,

and I'm Going to Teach You the L.A. Hustle...'

With the L.A. Hustle any number can play. It's not done with a partner, but with one or more (preferably a lot more) people all moving in the same direction, all doing the same step at the same time. Hopefully.

"The steps in this eight-count dance are highly choreographed, and the rest of the body's motion is highly stylized. Think strut: Swing your arms, with a lift in the shoulder and elbow. Try marching in place, swinging your arms and body from side to side—then play it down a little. When you do the steps, you should be swinging. Lift your knees and pick up your feet in a deliberate way; don't just shuffle.

"The dance breaks down into four parts: first backward and forward; then side to side; then short jumps topped off with a

---

Karen Lustgarten is a disco dance instructor in San Francisco.

chicken flap; and finally standing in place, poking around with your right toe—winding up with a kick, which leads into the first step of the set again.

"Beginning with your feet together, take three steps backward: Step back with the right foot, then back with the left foot, back with the right foot, then touch your left toe to the left side. Reverse direction, stepping forward on the left foot, forward on the right foot, forward on the left foot, and touch with the right foot. This should take you eight beats. Repeat this entire series walking back three steps, then touch forward three steps, then touch, so that steps 9 through 16 are the same as steps 1 through 8. Now you're ready for Phase Two, which begins moving to the right side.

"To do this, step to the right side with the right foot. Then cross your left foot in front of your right. Step to the right side again with your right foot, then touch your left foot to the left

1) **Phase One** (backward-forward-side-touch) begins with three steps backward, starting with the right foot. 2) A step to the side with the right foot starts **Phase Two** (side-to-side movements). 3) Another Phase Two position: Crossing the left foot in front of the right. 4) The last of Phase Two's four sideways steps: A touch to the left with the left foot after uncrossing your legs. 5) **Phase Three** (jumps, chicken flaps and heel clicks) starts with a jump forward and a pause.

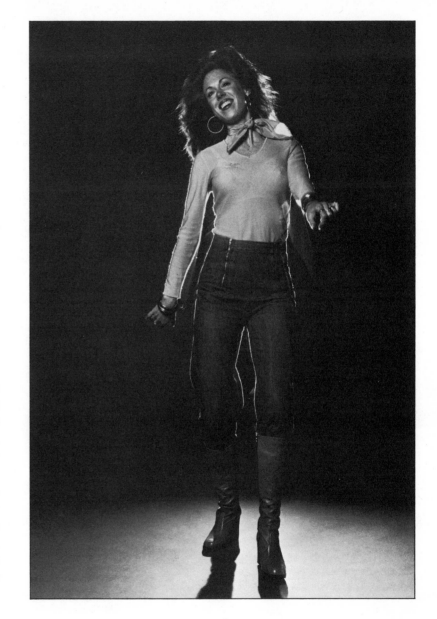

side. That's four beats. Now you reverse, moving to the left side: Step left with your left foot, cross right, step left and bring your right foot together with your left. Altogether that's eight beats (side, cross, side, touch; side, cross, side, step) which are not repeated. End of Phase Two, with your weight on your left foot.

"To begin Phase Three, jump forward and pause, then jump back and pause; then repeat the two jumps a bit faster. Now separate your heels and click them together. Do this twice. As your heels go out, your elbows do too, and as your heels click together, your elbows come in, chicken style. This sequence will be eight beats; jump up, pause, jump back, pause, jump up faster and pause, jump back faster and pause, click, click.

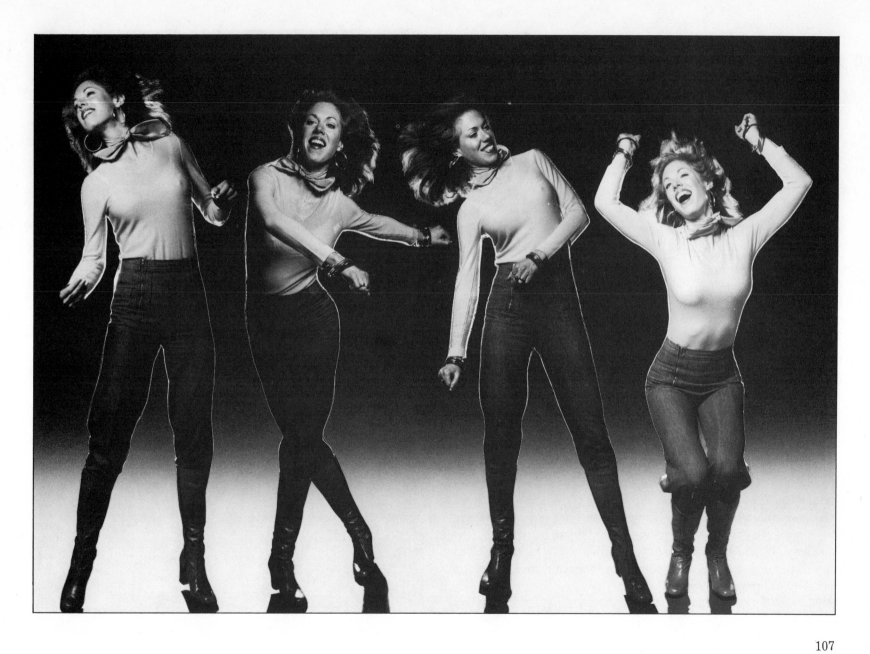

6) The first half of the chicken flap: Heels and elbows go out . . .
7) . . . and come back in, with heels clicking together. 8) The first
step of Phase Four (toe touching and the kick): Touching the
right foot to the front. 9) A quarter turn to the left and a kick
with the right foot: The grand finale of Phase Four. 10) Starting
over with Phase One: Ready to step back with the right.

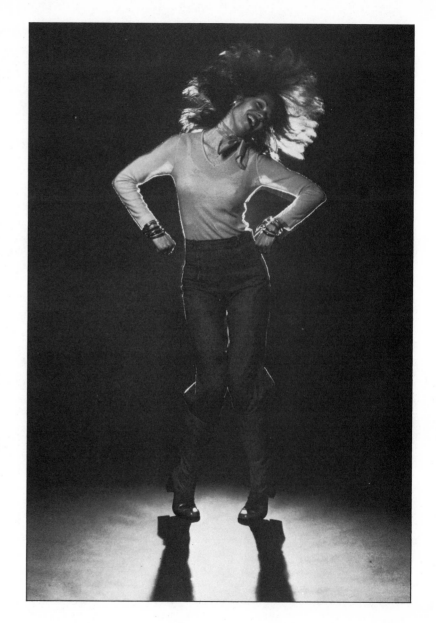

"For your last series of moves, touch your right foot out in
front of you two times, then touch your right foot behind you
two times. Then touch it once forward, once behind, once to
the side; then kick it across your left leg while you turn your
whole body (one-quarter turn) to the left. This sequence will
be eight beats: forward for two, back for two, forward, back,
side, kick. That right foot you've just kicked will now step back
and start the whole dance all over from step one, but facing
90° counterclockwise from where you started.

"Okay. That's the basic step. Remember that you can replace
any of the later phases with your own turns and jumps, so long
as they hold the eight-count time."

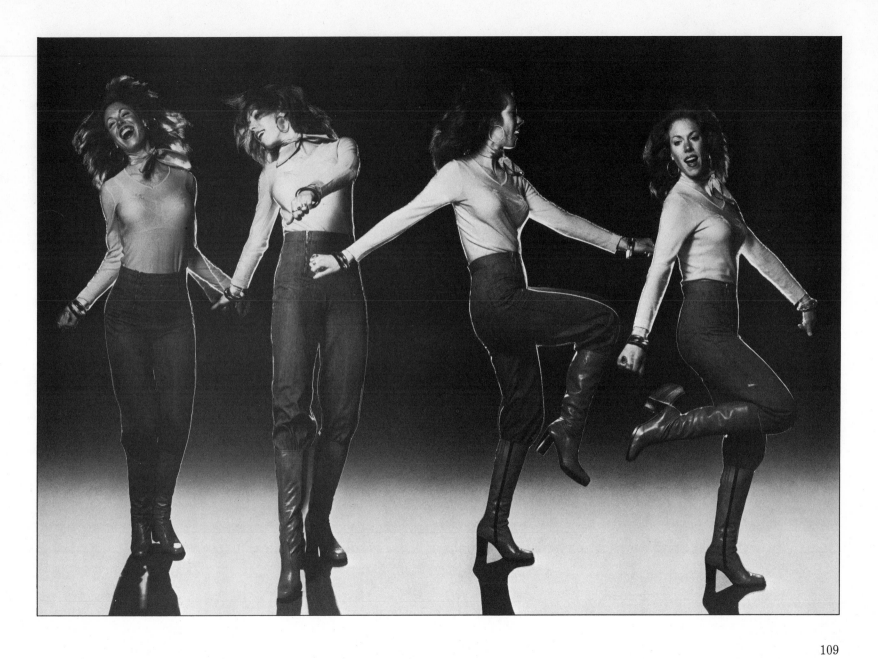

Like any good craze, the current disco boom has already provided lucrative hit-and-run windfalls for a wide assortment of profiteers—club owners, dance instructors, T-shirt makers, rock magazines—and we can probably expect new ones to start cashing in at any moment. For example, the medical profession.

That dark thought occurred to me the other night when I was introduced to a novel therapeutic discipline called *discogenics* by Dr. Gilbert J. Kucera, a handsome, 43-year-old orthopedic surgeon. Sitting in the lounge of a Bay Area disco, I began to suspect that Dr. Kucera was having sport with me. For one thing, I couldn't find any other physician who'd ever heard of discogenics. And Dr. Kucera himself apparently hadn't heard of it before inventing the term a few hours before our interview. "Has a nice sound to it, don't you think?" he said with a twinkle in his eye. Yet, seriously folks, Dr. Kucera recently has been treating a number of patients with swollen disks, minor "slipped" disks and general injuries of the lumbar region suffered after dancing too strenuously at discos not unlike the one we were visiting that very moment. And he has good credentials to analyze the problem. He knows about dancing because he's a dancer himself and once worked as an Arthur Murray instructor. He knows about young bodies because he is currently a medical adviser to the U.S. Olympic ski team.

"First let me emphasize that I think dancing is a very good body exercise," he said. "One of the best. People who dance most of their life stay young most of their life. But you have to do it regularly and progressively—a little at first, then more as your body gets looser. There's no question this puts a tremendous strain on your back. Some positions are real abnormal."

What happens, explained Dr. Kucera, is that when people get to be about 25, their disks start to degenerate. "Yes, it sounds awful, I know; my patients don't like me to tell them that. But that's exactly what happens. Those little cushions in

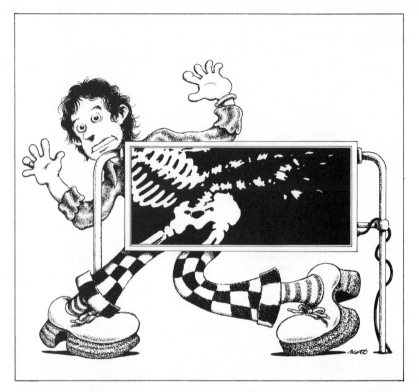

your spinal column start to get less pliable, more rigid." Which means that occasionally, when an aspiring but inexperienced disco dancer decides to bend way back or to the side in one of the most artistic, soulful and beautifully executed dance moves of his entire life, one of his disks may not go along with the idea. Instead it slips out of line, intrudes on the spinal nerves and produces a most powerful pain, causing the unfortunate victim to perform his next dance—the Hobble—on the way to Dr. Kucera's office.

"What do you do for these people?" I asked.

"I tell them to stop dancing. You know, get off your feet, go home and soak in a tub, stop dancing for a while. Usually this

SLIPPED DISCO

Out of Shape? Shoes Too Tight?
Beware of Things that Go Bump in the Night.
by David Felton

dancing causes only temporary injury—nothing permanent."

But certainly the sort of thing we'd all like to avoid. Therefore Dr. Kucera has obliged us with the following pointers:

• Warm up slowly, proceed with caution. This might include actual physical exercises, the kind you see real athletes do on television. Or a few nights of short dance sessions before you try an all-night howler.

• Cool off slowly. After dancing, take a warm shower or a Jacuzzi. Shy away from the cold night air.

• Stay loose—in mind and body. Whatever you need to accomplish this is all right with Dr. Kucera.

• Avoid excessive or extreme movements, particularly moving backward and twisting at the same time. In other words, avoid making an ass of yourself and you'll probably be okay.

• Wear loose shoes, wide shoes, flat shoes. This may not help your back, but it prevents blisters.

Dr. Kucera and I decided to check out the dance floor, which at that time was filled with some 60 writhing patrons dancing their asses off. Everyone seemed to enjoy it but, as Dr. Kucera indicated, some were certainly more demonstrative than others. The distinguished practitioner of discogenics scanned the floor with his professional eye, smiled and said, "There's gonna be a lot of sore backs tomorrow morning."

SECTION II

FIRST STEPS

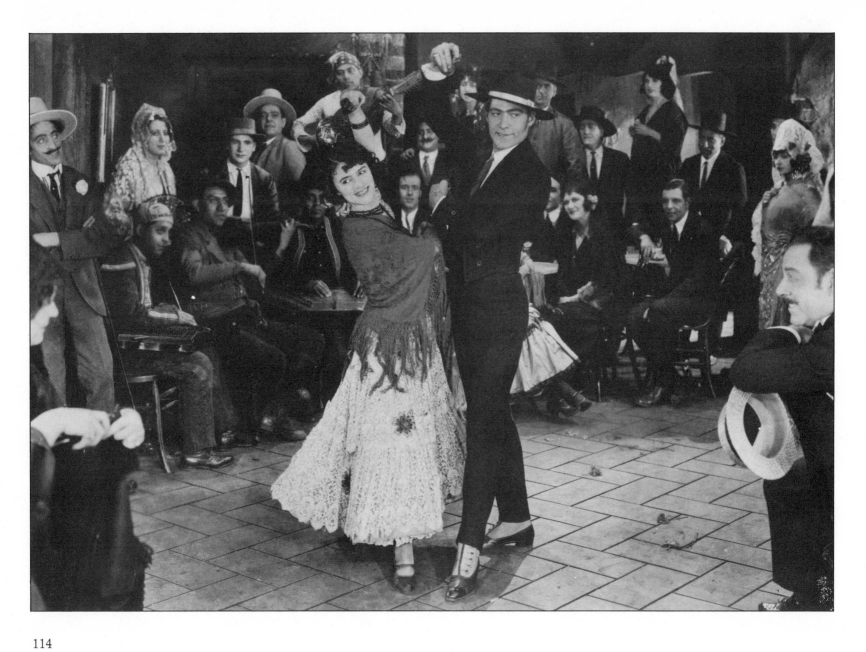

IT SEEMS WE'VE STOOD AND DANCED LIKE THIS BEFORE

Seven Decades of Dance

by Marshall Rosenthal

THE TURN OF THE CENTURY

To celebrate without dancing is like eating Oreos without milk. The taste is sweet but the wet exhilaration of a fundamental force washing the sweetness inward is missing. Dancing is a joyful, sexy activity, a people's art that reflects who we are and what we're up to.

At a wedding, the old folks Waltz and Tango and Fox Trot; the parents of the group Rumba and Charleston and Jitterbug; aunts and uncles call for the Cha-Cha, Mambo, Merengue and Twist; and "the kids" raise their arms in the air and move their bodies in any way that feels good, doing the Hustle, the Bump or the Woodstock Sungrope.

Remember Woodstock? A counterculture gathered in the 1969 mud of upstate New York to share Janis's singular blues and Jimi's personal, tortured vision of "The Star-Spangled Banner." It was a time of anarchistic social turmoil and those who chose to dance to the new anthem did so in their own space within the mob, hardly touching one another and following no prescribed set of steps.

John Philip Sousa wrote anthems too. His turn-of-the-century tunes were timed to the beat of the military tuba and the expansionist Spanish-American War. Americans did a jaunty Two Step to Sousa's "Washington Post March" and gave the brass-band leader scores of marching dance hits.

But young people have never been easily regimented, and dancing always has been the province of the young. As the new century opened in the New World, the fixed patterns of the American Two Step and the European 3/4 time Waltz gave way to African rhythms that put more spontaneity and sensuality into dance forms.

The Tango, a clearly sexual Argentinian dance whose origins have been traced to African slaves shipped to Cuba and Haiti in the early 1700s, swept post-Victorian, pre-World War I America. Its sinuous three-step-and-pause pattern was swiftly tamed and divorced from its raffish gypsy origins, and "Tango teas" became a pastime of the upper crust. Still, "imitate the sensuous grace of the tiger, mademoiselle" remained a Tango instruction of the day, and the sexual sullenness of Rudolph Valentino later came to personify the melancholy dance that Vernon and Irene Castle, America's best-known dance team, popularized on the vaudeville stage.

THE GREAT WAR

At the same time, American Negro jazz, with its syncopations and improvisations, had entered the mainstream. "Ragtime" (syncopated) music became thoroughly commercialized, with Irving Berlin's "Alexander's Ragtime Band" of 1911 being a middle-brow bow to the artistry of Scott Joplin and Jelly Roll Morton. The Turkey Trot, popularized by the Castles, was danced to the ragtime-tinged "Everybody's Doing It" in the 1913 Ziegfeld Follies.

That same Ziegfeld revue saw comedian Harry Fox take to the stage and do some trotting steps accompanied by ragtime music that one contemporary critic found to be "very rollicking," with "a tendency to put everyone in good humor." The dance became known as the Fox Trot, and its 4/4 rhythms are still with us as we wrap ourselves around our partners and do a slow, dreamy box step to a song by Andy Williams or Barbra Streisand, Kris Kristofferson or Paul Simon.

The years before "The Great Interruption," as the Duchess

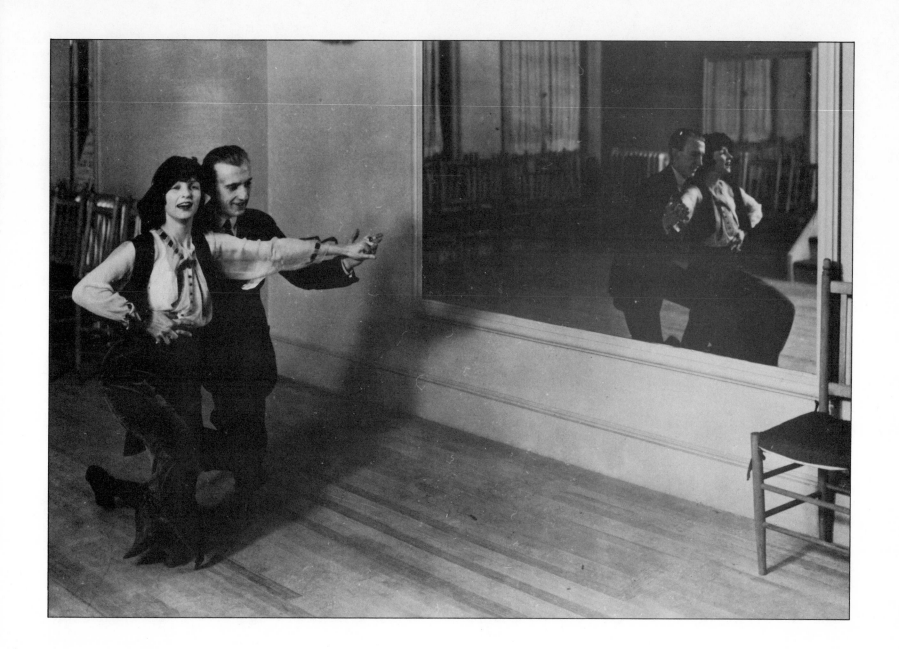

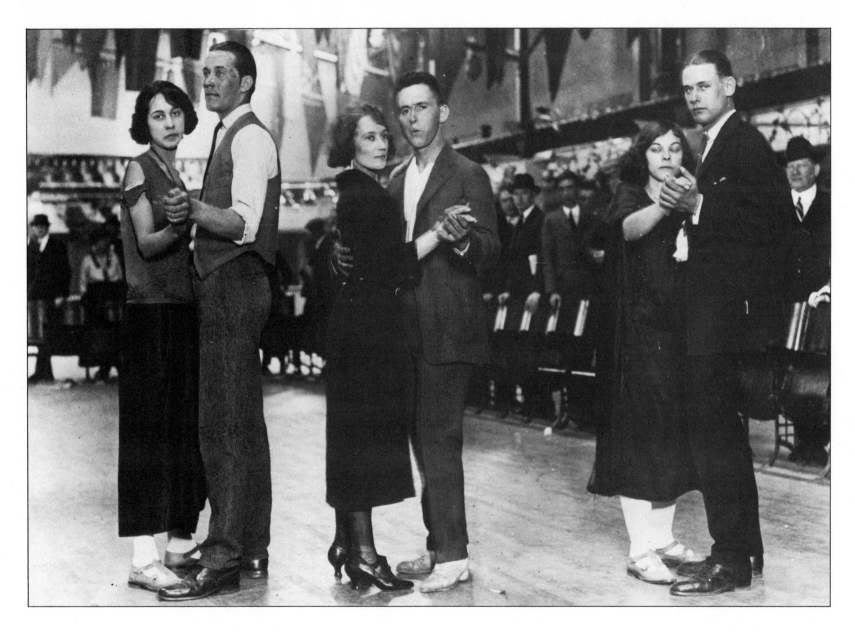

of Westminster graciously dubbed World War I, were most innovative for popular dancing. American popular music began to emphasize danceable rhythms at the expense of lyrics or even melody. Junior proms were born, and any restaurant that yearned for business had to provide a space for dancing. After the war, however, the dance hall gave way to the phonograph as the medium with the dance-music message. The cultural historian, Russell Nye, in his book *The Unembarrassed Muse: The Popular Arts in America* quotes a Twenties Victor ad as follows:

"You cannot resist dancing when the music is provided by His Master's Voice. The tunes . . . have a snap which only those famous dance orchestras that record for Victor can give them. *You can dance whenever you like.*" (Emphasis added.)

"For the next 50 years," Nye writes, "dancing—whether it be the Charleston, the Black Bottom, the Big Apple, the Lindy Hop or the Twist and Boogaloo—was inextricably linked with the record business and popular songs."

THE TWENTIES

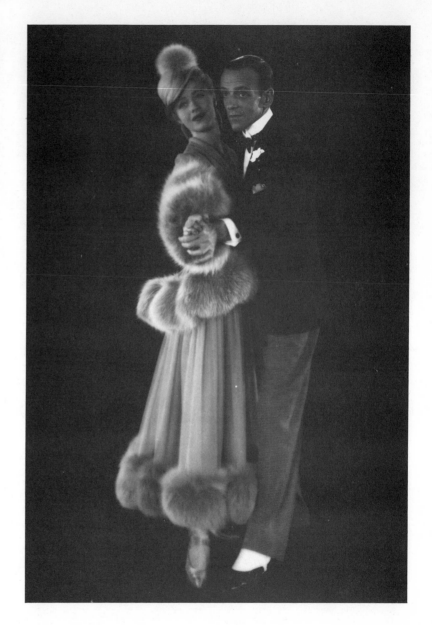

By the end of the war, the Protestant ethic was certainly wounded if not dead. Veterans returned from Over There with condoms in their pockets, and Henry Ford's automobile provided a spot to spark. Theda Bara was mostly bare in her popular silent films, and dancing had moved out of ballrooms and into intimate nightclubs and living rooms.

The Twenties was the period of Harding and Coolidge, Prohibition and the St. Valentine's Day Massacre. Europe still stumbled about—a putsch in Munich, a power struggle in Moscow—but in America it was Flappers and All That Jazz.

There was jazz for every dancing taste. Hot jazz trumpeted "Runnin' Wild," Guy Lombardo's Royal Canadians played "the sweetest music this side of heaven," and Paul Whiteman's "symphonic jazz" reached its peak in a 1924 concert when Whiteman featured George Gershwin at the piano in his own *Rhapsody in Blue*.

Dancing teachers in the Twenties still found "ladies and gentlemen" who wanted to learn the Fox Trot, the Boston (a variety of Waltz) and the One-Step (a faster predecessor of the Fox Trot); but the shakings, embracings and contortions of the vulgar Flapper dances—the Shimmy, the Charleston and the Black Bottom, Negro dances all—scandalized much of polite society and were not taught in proper dancing schools.

The story may be apocryphal, but the Charleston is said to have originated with blacks in Charleston, South Carolina, who were parodying the dancing of white debutantes. Whatever its origin, the Charleston made it into a 1923 Broadway musical and swept the country in 1924 via films and phonograph records. A few years later came the bouncy Lindy Hop, created at Harlem's Savoy Ballroom in honor of Charles Lindbergh's solo flight across the Atlantic in 1927. Eventually it assumed an easily teachable beat but, like the Charleston, it retained much of its open sexuality and room for individual expression.

THE THIRTIES

Enter the Thirties and enter Depression. The Rumba, a Cuban import, was the big dance of the new decade in cafe society. The temper of the time is recaptured in Thomas Parson's *How to Dance* manual: "The Rumba is a nonprogressive dance, with couples dancing in relatively small areas rather than making progress around the floor. As a consequence, one of the first items of study is to learn to take small steps and to *stay in your own square!* . . . Anyone can learn how to do this."

Spontaneous New Orleans-style jazz faded in the Thirties, to be replaced with big band swing. Characterized in part by repetitive phrases (called "riffs") and solo improvisations played over tightly written ensemble arrangements, it was a less frenzied sound than New Orleans jazz, but a very danceable one with a pronounced "big beat." Again, the watchword of the day was "regularization," and people got what they wanted.

The Bennie Goodman and the Jimmie and Tommy Dorsey dance bands may have grossed a half-million dollars a year—during the Depression. There were more than 300 big bands with a national reputation, and dance broadcasts—second in popularity only to comedians among radio listeners—beamed across America from "high atop the Hotel Ansonia in beautiful downtown . . ." Decca Records, organized in 1934, specialized in 35¢ dance records, an increasing number of which began to wind up, not on home record players, but in jukeboxes and the libraries of radio stations. It was the golden age of the film musical—and maybe the golden age of popular music in America.

And if a fellow couldn't spare a dime to take his gal dancing, he could take her to Marathon dance contests to watch other bozos play out his fantasies on the dance floor. *They Shoot Horses, Don't They?* dramatized the agonies of the Marathon; the truth was even more devastating.

According to the *Guinness Book of World Records,* "The most severe Marathon (staged as a public spectacle in the U.S.) was one lasting 3780 hours (22 weeks, 3½ days). This was completed by Callum L. De Villier, now of Minneapolis, and Miss Vonnie Kuchinski in Somerville, Massachusetts, from December 28, 1932, to June 3, 1933. In the last two weeks the

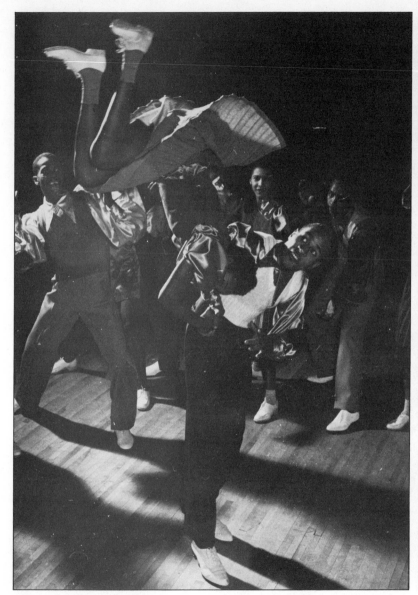
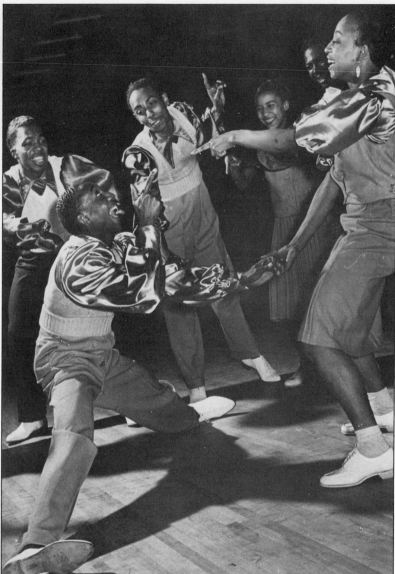

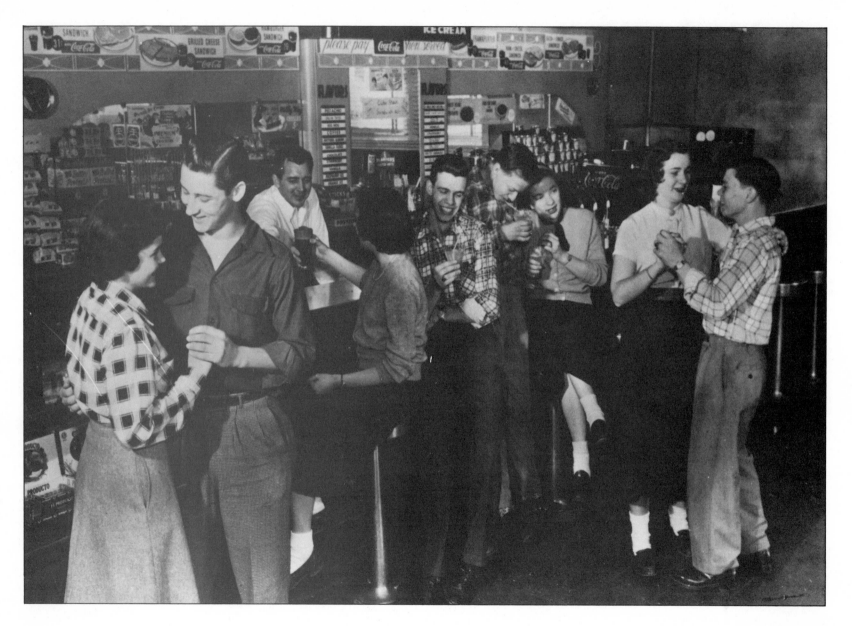

rest allowance was cut from 15 minutes per hour to only three minutes while the last 52½ hours were continuous. The prize of $1000 was equivalent to less than 26½¢ per hour."

Nevertheless, the Samba, a joyful Brazilian carnival dance introduced at the 1939 New York World's Fair, became popular in the U.S. through the movie musicals of Carmen Miranda. This uptempo variation of the Fox Trot vied for dance band attention with the Conga, a Latin dance imported from the pre-jet Jet Set of the French Riviera. The Conga was most in tune with the regimen which had been the Thirties. A roomful of dancers formed a line, each placing their hands on the hips of the person in front of them, and while the Latin rhythms played, the dancers followed the leader anywhere, or nowhere.

THE FORTIES

The Forties opened with a hot war and closed with a cold one. During World War II, dancing was curtailed in Germany; it provided a release in war-torn England, and in America, with a great number of its men in the armed forces, everyone made do with the materials at hand.

This was the leanest decade of dance innovation. The Jitterbug, a fast and furious swing-band dance, was popularized in England by the GIs—not without shocking some by its "vulgar and uninhibited movements." Nevertheless, the zoot-suited men at home in their broad-shouldered pin-striped jackets, baggy-kneed pants and key chains that hooked on to the waistband, looped to the pegged cuff and returned to the pocket, persisted in athletically lifting, twisting and spinning their Jitterbug partners about.

By 1945, however, the swing era was over. The draft, gas rationing, amusement taxes, midnight curfews and sloppy playing by those who'd enjoyed a bonanza staying Stateside spelled the end of swing, and most musicians found work only in recording studios or with smaller bands fronted by vocalists like Frank Sinatra, Dinah Shore, Ella Fitzgerald, Perry Como or Tony Bennett.

Jazz moved to Bop, developed by Charlie Parker and Dizzy Gillespie, and Bop, with its complex rhythms and intricate harmonics, did not move folks to dance.

The Mambo, a musical combination of Afro-Cuban rhythms and progressive jazz, was the major new dance of the Forties. It was similar in form to the Samba: Dancing partners still held one another, with the male partner showing the way. As with other dances, the wild, primitive Mambo was soon standardized into a syncopated rhythm more easily mastered by postwar dance fans.

THE FIFTIES

On television, dance-studio owners Arthur and Kathryn Murray urged viewers to "put a little fun in your life—try dancing." Such fun, in the form of the Murrays' "Lifetime Executive Course," could cost $12,000, but would certainly prepare anybody to dance to the "grown-up" music of Eddie Fisher, Perry Como or Harry Belafonte. Belafonte's RCA album, *Calypso*, was one of the first LPs to sell a million copies.

Like the Thirties, this decade of readjustment opened with low-key, sophisticated dances. The Merengue, which could be danced to Samba music but required less dexterity, was imported from the Caribbean and, in its early version, called for dancers to take a sideward left step, then *drag* the right foot

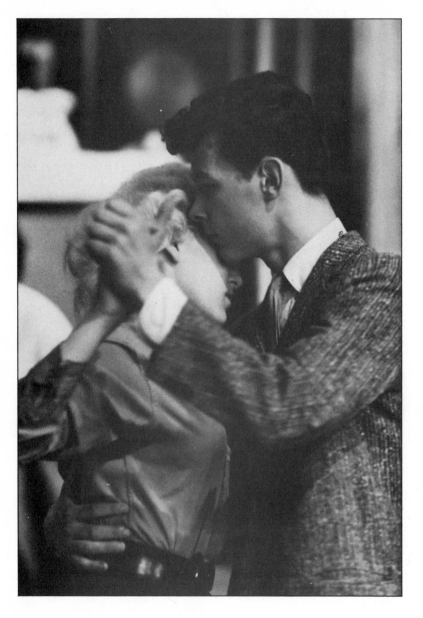

toward the left. Legend had it that the dance originated when a crippled Dominican Republic military leader danced at an official ball and the guests respectfully followed his lead as he dragged his lame right leg.

The Cha-Cha, a Cuban dance which grew out of the Mambo, was the smash of the mid-Fifties. Its unique triple step (cha-cha-cha) was easily learned, and there were plenty of twists and turns for individual expression. Perez Prado had a top-selling Cha-Cha single in 1955 with "Cherry Pink and Apple Blossom White."

The Number One record of 1955, however, was "Rock around the Clock" by Bill Haley and the Comets. It created a revolution, and New York disc jockey Alan Freed coined the phrase "rock 'n' roll"—picking it up from sexual blues lyrics of the Twenties like "My baby rocks me with one steady roll"—in order to classify the new music emerging from black rhythm & blues artists like Chuck Berry and Fats Domino.

Besides records, radio and the movies, rock 'n' roll exploded onto the newest mass medium, television. Elvis Presley made three high-priced, above-the-waist appearances on *The Ed Sullivan Show* in 1956 and early 1957, and a prim, short-haired Philadelphia disc jockey, Dick Clark, brought his *American Bandstand* show to network television. Teens all over the country rushed home from school to watch clean-cut Elvis imitators like Fabian and Frankie Avalon "lipsynch" their hits and dance along as regulars like Justine Corelli and Kenny Rossi did the Stroll, the Chicken and the Fish.

But the dance that broke into the mainstream was the Twist. The Twist was the first big disco dance in that it involved an opposite, walking movement, coordinating, say, the left leg and the right arm. Only instead of walking, everyone was Twisting.

"The Twist had no orderly series of steps, a peculiarly sexless avoidance of bodily contact," Russel Nye writes, "and it left the individual freedom to move as he wished. The Twist

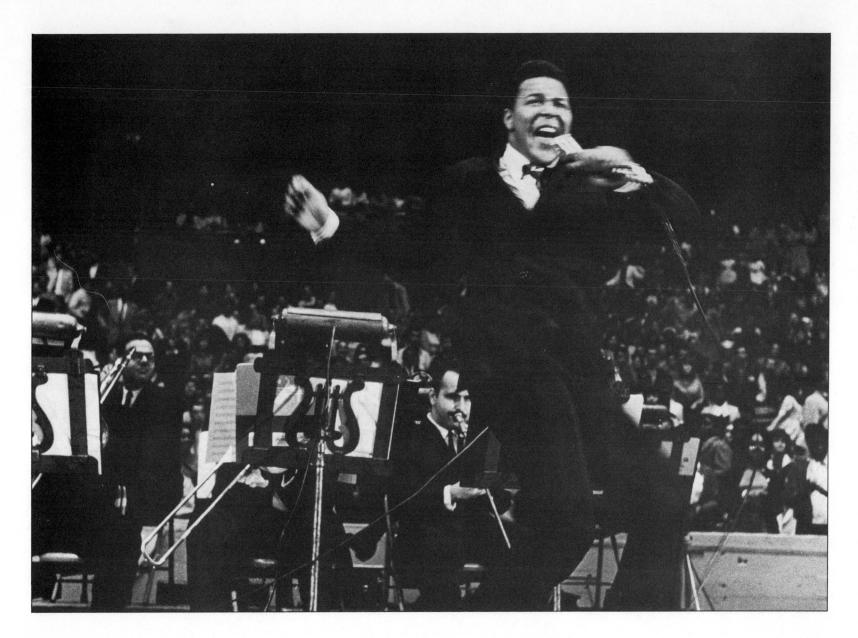

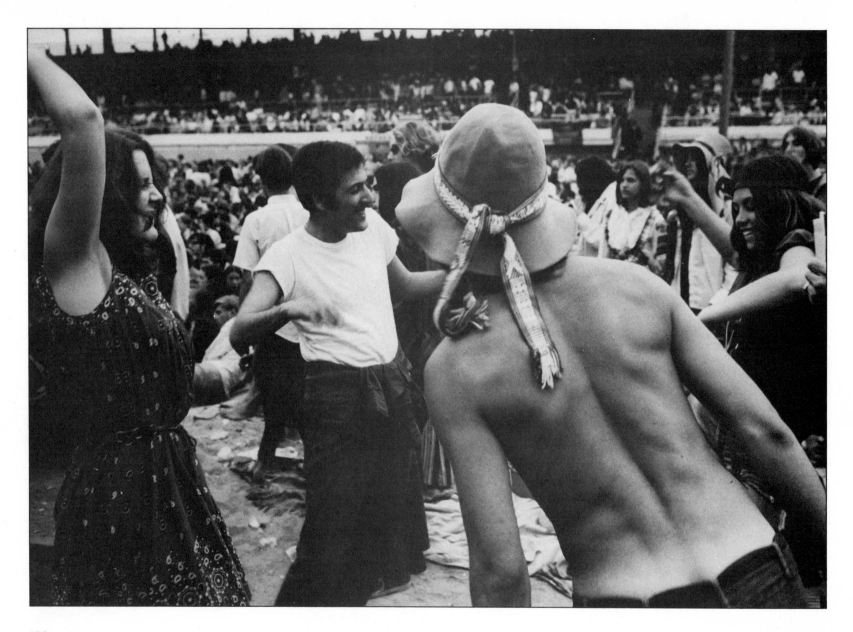

was easy to do and mildly daring—not enough to get high school students ejected from Saturday night dances; simple enough for the white nightclub trade."

The Twist was a safe dance for a safe time. It was accompanied by a crude form of popular music, and couples wooed one another with glances rather than touches.

THE SIXTIES

Though the Twist had no steps to it, some pattern dances became popular in the Sixties. The Watusi combined the one-two-three bounce motion of the Pony with the body motion of the Twist; the white version of this dance done outside the West Coast updated the side-cross pattern of the Conga and transformed the Watusi into a line dance where teens of opposite sexes faced each other and clapped their hands to a rock & roll cadence. The Pony itself was a white favorite because the girls could feel their hair move freely as they shook it to the beat.

There were others. The Boogaloo was a step-and-tap couple dance, which became the Funky Broadway when partners bent their knees on even counts. The Slop and the Mashed Potato were black-originated dances that stressed style more than the simple steps. But whether a dance involved recognizable foot patterns, like the Skate, the swivel motions of the Frug or the up-and-down bobbings of the Philly Dog, the Sixties continued the trend away from touching. The Jerk involved putting a hand over your head and snapping your body so that an arm would rapidly descend. The Monkey was another up-and-down dance built around imaginary tree-climbing. The aptly named Hitchhike didn't even bother with leg movement. Perhaps the most ridiculous dance spawned by the thousands of discos, shows, movies and parties was the Clam, a dance from an Elvis movie called *Girls! Girls! Girls!* in which the women bent over as if they were digging up clams. It bombed.

During the early Sixties, people celebrated the spirit of Camelot by dancing at parties and discotheques. Discos like the Peppermint Lounge and Arthur attracted jet-setters like Liz and Dick and professional dancers like Killer Joe Piro; lesser-known spots were havens for kids who'd spent the night before at the drive-in. Chubby Checker and Bobby Freeman (who still does his act at a topless nightclub in San Francisco) exhorted one and all to do the Twist and the Swim. As a song by a group called Cannibal & the Headhunters said in its title, it was a "land of a thousand dances."

As the decade progressed, the advent of rock, which accented the up beat, led to an even less structured kind of dancing among the young whites who were coming to be called "Hippies." Young blacks stuck to heavily accented soul music, but their long-haired counterparts explored the stranger off rhythms of acid rock. Music became a social ritual, and the rock festival replaced the disco, which went the way of the pool hall and the Hula Hoop. By the time we got to Woodstock, dancing was a formless expression of ecstacy instead of a structured sequence of steps.

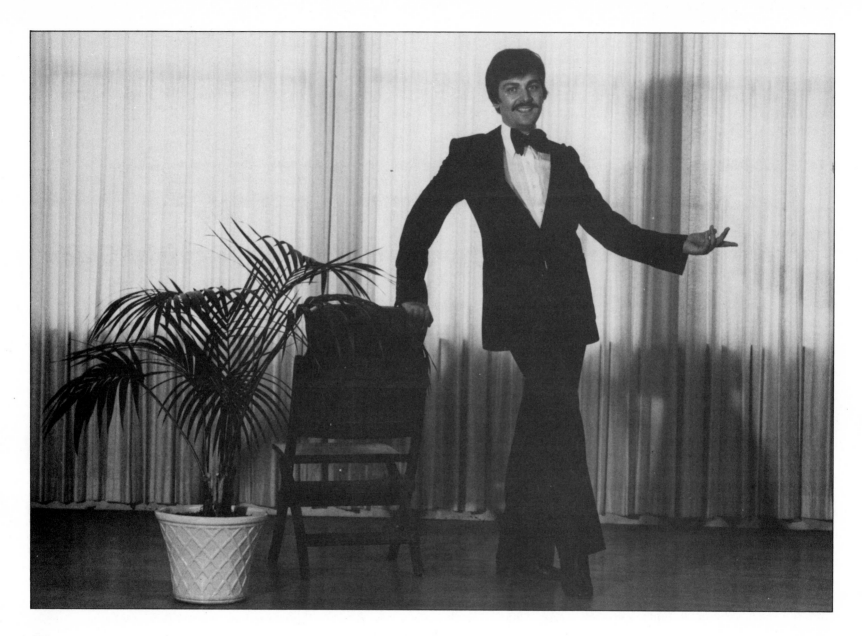

128

"HI, I'M TEDDY LEE

and Here's the Wedding/Prom/Bar Mitzvah Survival Guide

It's a common problem. You're at a family affair or a local social, and the men in the Guy Lombardo Band suits strike up some dance you've never learned. And then, who appears but your battle-ax aunt or a pasty in-law with an invitation to trip the light fantastic out on the dance floor. What to do?

Meet Teddy Lee, Pro Dancer, master of those steps that have withstood the test of time and the man with the solution to your dilemma. Teddy Lee has won dance competitions in the Rumba, Samba, Paso Doble and Cha-Cha. He currently teaches dancing at his Renaissance School of Dance in San Francisco, and he's stripped down his instructions to provide the bare-bones steps necessary for your survival as a social guerrilla, be it at a wedding, prom or any other ceremonial occasion.

"Remember, dancing is moving your body with feeling in a well-coordinated manner harmonious to the music. In order to move your body to music, you should be aware of the rhythm and be able to count that rhythm." So get ready to count, and let Teddy and Ingrid show you how to hold your own.

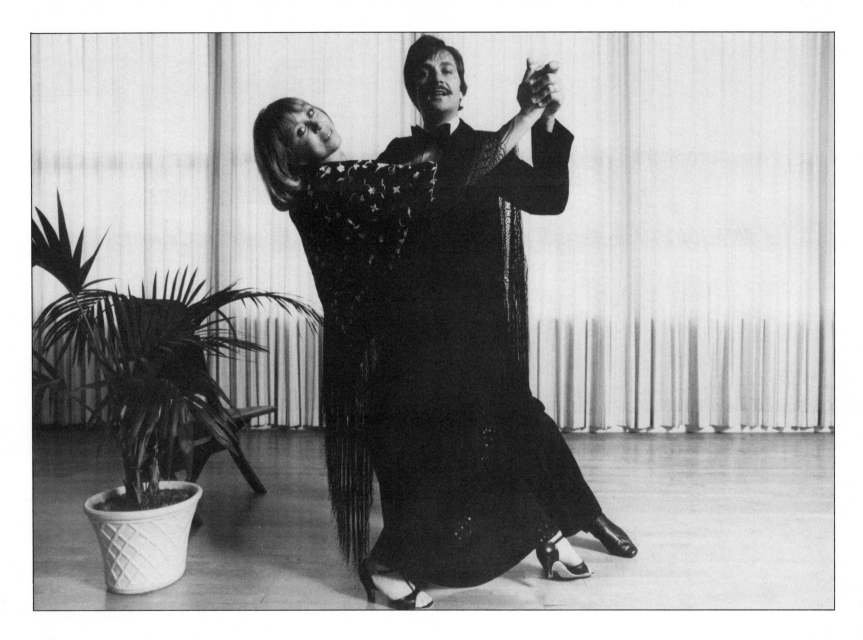

THE FOX TROT

"While We're Out Together Dancing Cheek to Cheek"

The quick trot that Harry Fox previewed on the Ziegfeld stage was refined through Vern and Irene Castle and others into a smoother, slower, more streamlined dance. Now the Fox Trot is danced everywhere, with a slow, medium or medium-fast tempo.

"Since there are only three steps and the Fox Trot is a four-count dance, one of the steps counts for two beats. This is the slow step. The basic rhythm we're teaching you to follow is slow-quick-quick. Step on the first beat and slide the other foot on the second without shifting your weight. Then, when you take two quick steps, you'll have danced to four beats.

"The Fox Trot is danced in Social Dance Position: Partners face each other, his arm lightly touching her at the waist. The woman's left hand rests on the man's upper arm near his shoulder, and their other hands are clasped and extended to the side. Once in this position, a good basic step for the Fox Trot is the box step. A basic box step is done with one slow step and two quick steps to the count of one-two-three-four, and then repeated starting with the opposite feet. You'll notice that for the woman, the pattern is the opposite of the man's; she is doing the second part first and the first part second.

"Once you have the basic box step under control, you may want to branch out a little. Some possible patterns are the glide (a straightahead two-step), a six-beat pattern and the twinkle (a crossover step in Promenade Position—where the man and women's feet form a V). For simplicity's sake, we'll restrict our patterns to the box step and twinkle, danced to a slow-quick-quick rhythm."

131

FOX TROT
Boxstep

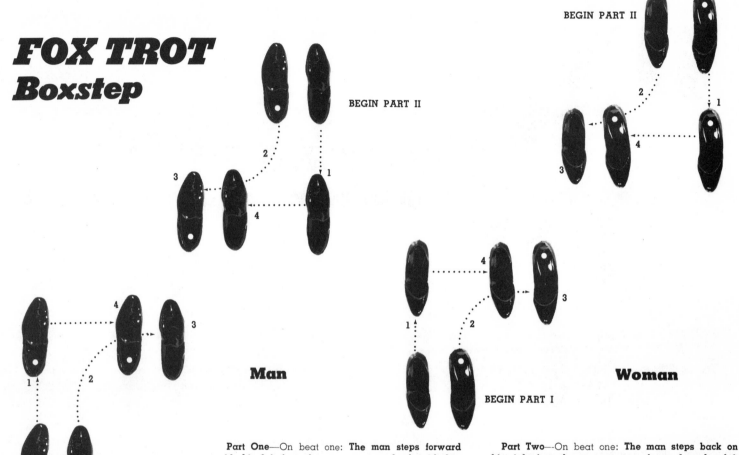

BEGIN PART II

BEGIN PART II

Man

Woman

BEGIN PART I

BEGIN PART I

Note: The left feet are marked with white dots

Part One—On beat one: **The man steps forward with his left foot, the woman steps back with her right foot.** On the beat two: **The man moves his right foot toward his left foot while keeping his weight on his left foot, the woman moves her left foot toward her right foot while keeping her weight on her right foot.** On beat three: **The man steps to his right side with his right foot, the woman steps to her left side with her left foot.** On beat four: **The man closes his left foot to his right foot and shifts weight, the woman closes her right foot to her left foot and shifts weight.**

Part Two—On beat one: **The man steps back on his right foot, the woman steps forward on her left foot.** On beat two: **The man moves his left foot toward his right foot while keeping his weight on his right foot, the woman moves her right foot toward her left foot while keeping her weight on her left foot.** On beat three: **The man steps to his left side with his left foot, the woman steps to her right side with her right foot.** On beat four: **The man closes his right foot to his left foot and shifts weight, the woman closes her left foot to her right and shifts weight.**

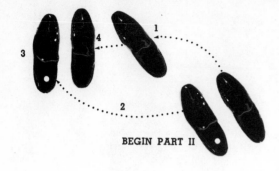

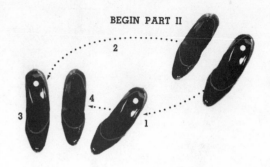

FOX TROT
Twinkle

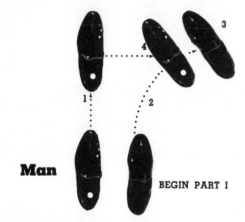

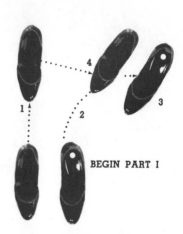

Man   BEGIN PART I

Woman   BEGIN PART I

Part One—On beat one: **The man steps forward with his left foot, the woman steps backward with her right foot.** On beat two: **The man moves his right foot toward his left foot while keeping his weight on his left foot, the woman moves her left foot toward her right foot while keeping her weight on her right foot.** On beat three: **The man moves his right foot to his right side with a slight turn to his left, the woman moves her left foot to her left side with a slight turn to her right.** On beat four: **The man closes his left foot to his right foot and changes weight, the woman

closes her right foot to her left foot and changes weight.**

Part Two—On beat one: **The man steps forward and slightly across his left foot with his right foot, the woman steps forward and slightly across her right foot with her left foot.** On beat two: **The man moves his left foot toward his right foot while keeping his weight on his right foot, the woman moves her right foot toward her left foot while keeping her weight on her left foot.** On beat three: **The man steps to his left side on his left foot, having turned slightly

to the right to face his partner, the woman steps to her right side on her right foot, having turned slightly to the left to face her partner.** On beat four: **The man closes his right foot to his left foot and changes weight, the woman closes her left foot to her right foot and changes weight.**

133

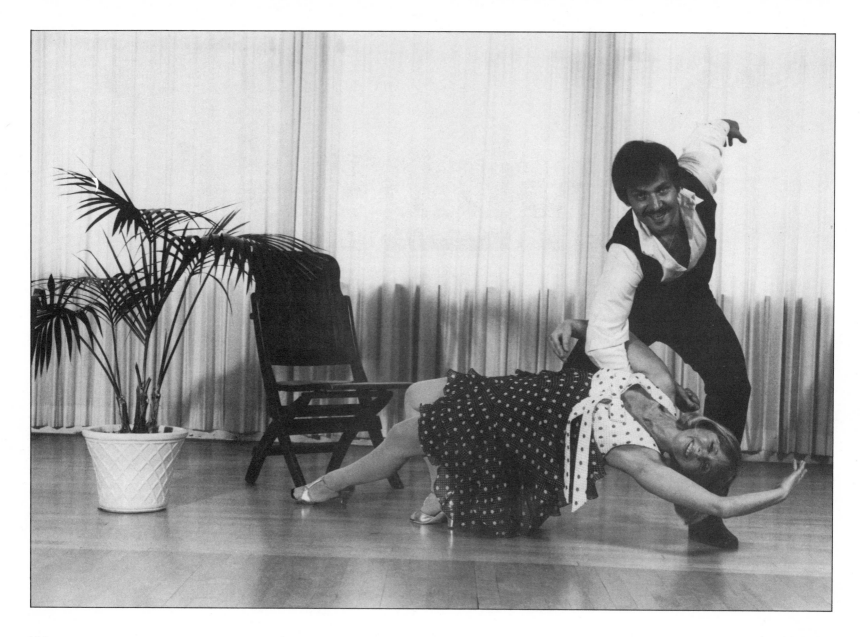

SWING

"It Don't Mean a Thing if It Ain't Got that Swing"

Swing is a fast dance. Its predecessors were the Lindy and the Jitterbug; later came be-bop and rock & roll dances. Although the original Lindy was an eight-beat dance, most teachers teach a six-beat step for Swing and Lindy. We'll teach the popular six-beat basic Swing, but please note that many advanced dancers use an eight-beat pattern whether they're dancing Swing or Lindy.

"You'll be doing eight steps to six beats of music. Think of the rhythm of this basic pattern as slow (rock)/slow(roll)/fast-fast/slow/fast-fast/slow to the count of one through six. Again, fast-fast means that these two steps take a total of one beat to complete. The Fox Trot accents its first and third beats; Swing is similar to rock & roll in that it accents its second and fourth beats.

"You may hold your partner in Social Dance Position, as well as in the Open Position [facing your partner and holding one or both of your partner's hands]. As they dance, Swing partners move toward and away from one another to the beat, swinging their upper bodies back and forth or from side to side.

"Turning moves are essential to Swing, and the basic Swing pattern may be done turning to the left or right. Another essential is the arch, or underarm turn, in which the man turns his partner under his upraised arm. Generally, though, the woman is doing a mirror image of what the man is doing—when he steps back with his left foot, she steps back with her right foot and so forth.

"Like the box step in Fox Trot, basic Swing may be danced continuously if you can't think of another step. But you should feel free to improvise, using the underarm turn in combination with the basic step and various pushaway or breakaway motions, in which partners step back and away from each other."

SWING
Basic

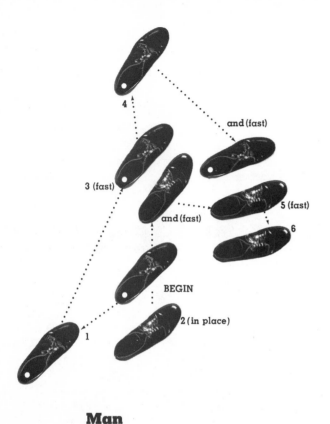

Man

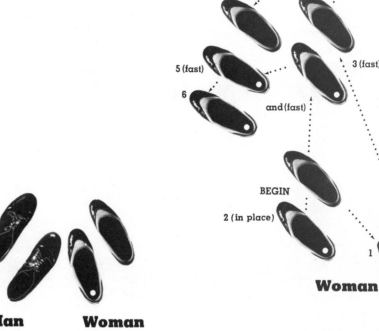

Woman

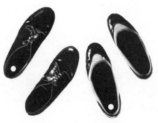

Man   **Woman**

PROMENADE POSITION

Note: The left feet are marked with white dots

On beat one: **From Promenade Position the man steps back on his left foot, the woman steps back on her right foot (rock).** On beat two: **The man picks up his right foot and puts it down in the same place, the woman picks up her left foot and puts it down in the same place (roll).** On beat three (count three and): **The man steps to his left side and forward with his left foot, closing his right foot toward his left, the woman steps to her right side and slightly forward with her right foot, closing her left foot toward her right (fast fast).** On beat four: **The man steps to his left side with his left foot, the woman steps to her right side with her right foot.** On beat five (count five and): **The man steps to his right side with his right foot and closes his left foot toward his right, the woman steps to her left side with her left foot and closes her right foot toward her left (fast fast).** On beat six: **The man steps to his right side with his right foot, the woman steps to her left side with her left foot.**

SWING
Underarm Turn

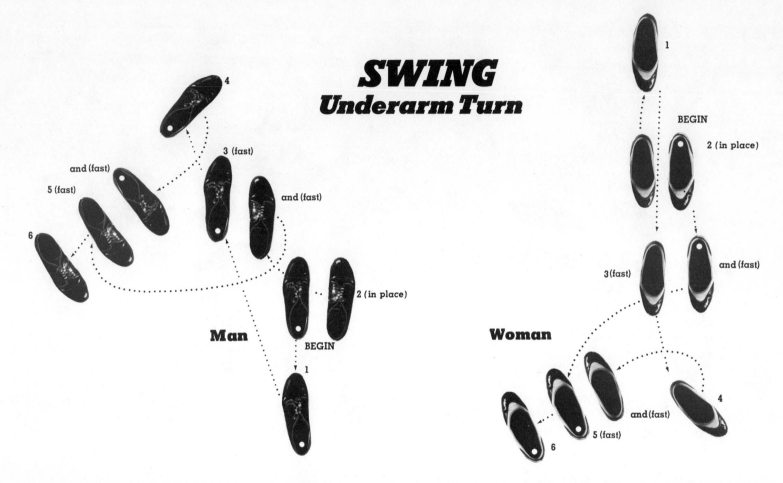

Man

Woman

Feel brave? On five and six of the basic step, the man lets go of his partner with his right hand, and the partners move away slightly with his left hand in her right hand. It's time for the underarm turn.

On beat one: While holding his partner's right hand with his left hand, the man steps back on his left foot, the woman steps back on her right foot (rock). On beat two: The man picks up his right foot and puts it down in the same place, the woman picks up her left foot and puts it down in the same place (roll). On beat

three (count three and): While lifting his partner's right hand in his left hand, the man steps forward and slightly to the left with his left foot, closing his right foot to his left foot while gently leading the woman to step forward on her right foot. The woman closes her left foot toward her right (fast fast). On beat four: **The man steps forward on his left foot toward the woman's right side, the woman steps forward on her right foot to the man's right side and turns under his raised left arm to her left.** On beat five (count five

and): The man moves his right foot backward and to the right and moves his left foot toward his right, the woman moves her left foot to her left side and closes her right foot toward her left (fast fast). On beat six: The man steps to his right side on his right foot to end facing his partner, the woman steps to her left side on her left foot to end facing her partner.

At this point, partners may resume the Social Dance Position and dance the basic step or they may stay in the Open Position and repeat the underarm turn.

137

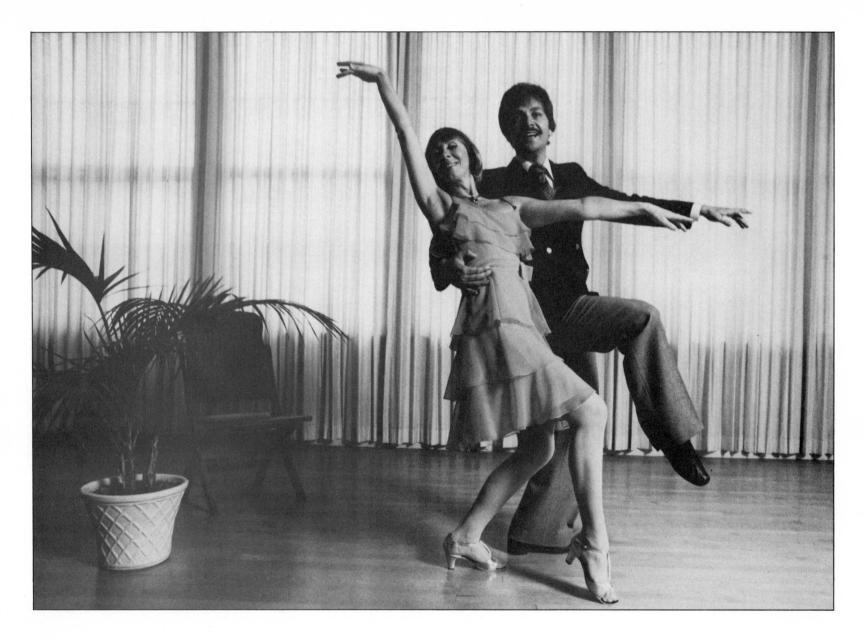

THE CHA-CHA

"It's Cherry Pink and Apple Blossom Time"

The Cha-Cha is a slower version of the Cuban Mambo or Latin salsa dances. In Cuba, when the Mambo was slowed down, the dancers became aware of a slightly syncopated sound played on the conga drum occurring on the fourth beat. This was called 'triple-beat Mambo,' and had a rhythm of one-two-three-boom-boom, and it became known as the Cha-Cha. Originally the dancers only moved their hips on the boom-boom [cha-cha], but later they began to move their feet as well.

"In slow-quick parlance, the Cha-Cha rhythm is slow-slow-slow-quick-quick.

"The steps we'll teach you are the basic Cha-Cha pattern and a side-to-side pattern with a break to the back. This step is also called a "fall-away break."

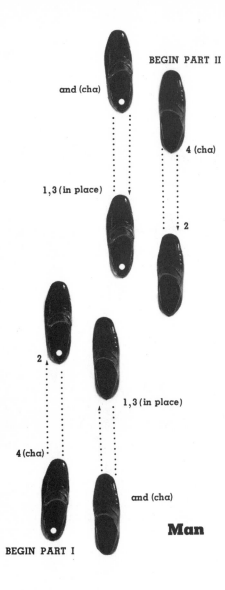

BEGIN PART II

and (cha)

4 (cha)

1,3 (in place)

2

2

1,3 (in place)

4 (cha)

and (cha)

Man

BEGIN PART I

CHA-CHA
Basic

"Here's a basic Cha-Cha: With left foot slightly ahead of the right, counting two measures of one, two, three, four and."

Part One—On beat one: **The man steps forward on his right foot, the woman steps backward on her left foot.** On beat two: **The man steps forward on his left foot, the woman steps backward on her right foot.** On beat three: **The man picks up his right foot and puts it down in the same place, the woman picks up her left foot and puts it down in the same place.** On four (count four and): **The man steps back quickly left-right, counting four and or cha-cha, the woman steps forward quickly right-left, counting four and or cha-cha.**

Part Two—On beat one: **The man steps back on his left foot, the woman steps forward on her right foot.** On beat two: **The man steps back on his right foot, the woman steps forward on her left foot.** On beat three: **The man picks up his left foot and puts it down in the same place, the woman picks up her right foot and puts it down in the same place.** On beat four (count four and): **The man steps forward quickly, right-left (cha-cha), the woman steps backward quickly, left-right (cha-cha).**

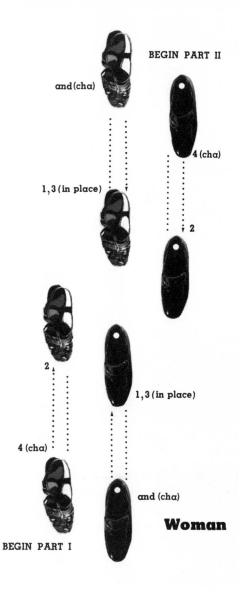

BEGIN PART II

and (cha)

4 (cha)

1,3 (in place)

2

2

1,3 (in place)

4 (cha)

and (cha)

Woman

BEGIN PART I

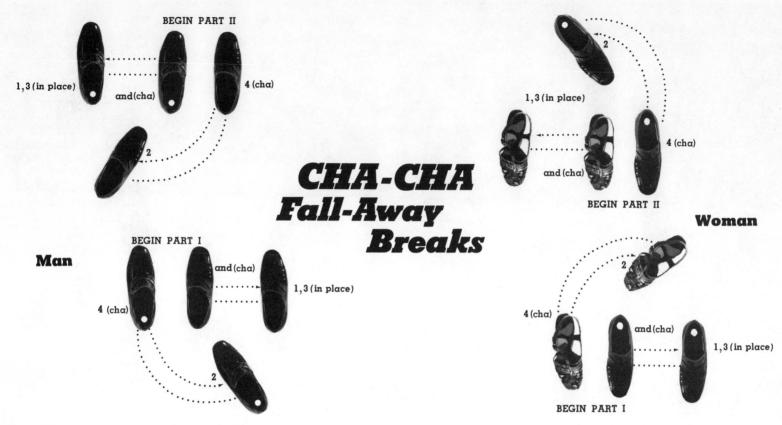

BEGIN PART II

1,3 (in place) and (cha) 4 (cha)

2

CHA-CHA
Fall-Away
Breaks

BEGIN PART I

and (cha) 1,3 (in place)

4 (cha)

2

Man

BEGIN PART II

2

1,3 (in place) 4 (cha)

and (cha)

BEGIN PART II

Woman

2

4 (cha) and (cha) 1,3 (in place)

BEGIN PART I

For something different, the Cha-Cha may be danced sideways instead of forward and backward. On four (count four and): The man steps right on his right foot and closes his left foot toward his right instead of cha-cha-ing forward. The woman steps on her left foot and closes her right foot toward her left instead of cha-cha-ing backward. Then . . .

Part One—On beat one: The man steps to his right side on his right foot, the woman steps to her left side on her left foot. On beat two: The man steps back on his left foot turning up to a quarter-turn left, the woman steps back on her right foot turning to her right. On beat three: The man picks up his right foot

and puts it down in the same place, the woman picks up her left foot and puts it down in the same place. On beat four (count four and): The man steps to his left side with his left foot and closes his right foot toward his left foot (cha-cha), the woman steps to her right side with her right foot and closes her left foot toward her right foot (cha-cha).

Part Two—On beat one: The man steps to his left side on his left foot, releasing his partner with his right hand, the woman steps to her right side on her right foot. On beat two: The man steps back on his right foot turning up to one-quarter turn to his right, the woman steps back on her left foot turning

up to one-quarter turn to her left. On beat three: The man picks up his left foot and puts it down in the same place, the woman picks up her right foot and puts it down in the same place. On beat four (count four and): Partners turn to face one another and return to Social Dance Position while the man steps to his right side with his right foot and closes his left foot toward his right foot (cha-cha), the woman steps to her left side with her left foot and closes her right foot toward her left (cha-cha).

This pattern may be repeated from beat one of the first part, or partners may return to the basic cha-cha. cha.

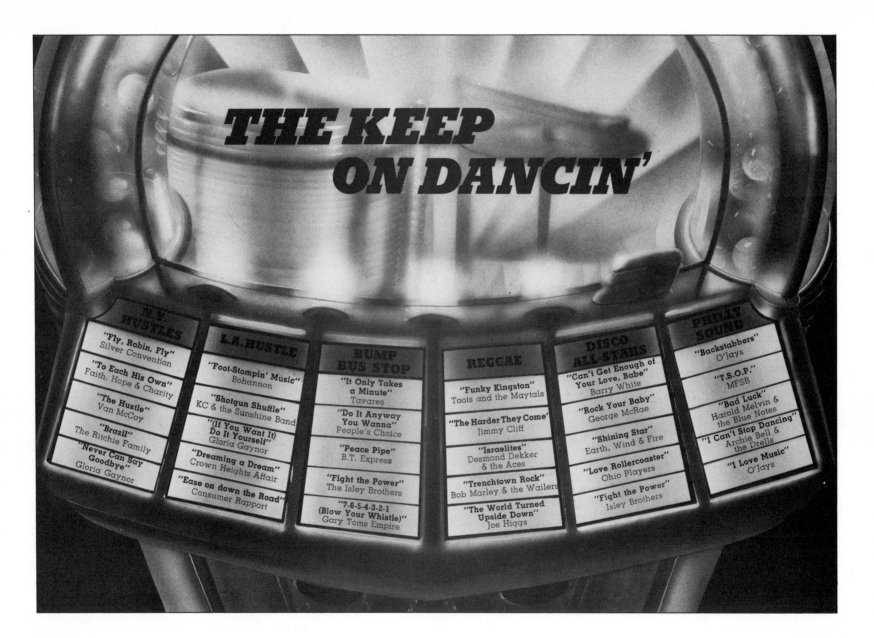

THE KEEP
ON DANCIN'

N.Y. HUSTLES

"Fly, Robin, Fly"
Silver Convention

"To Each His Own"
Faith, Hope & Charity

"The Hustle"
Van McCoy

"Brazil"
The Ritchie Family

"Never Can Say Goodbye"
Gloria Gaynor

L.A. HUSTLE

"Foot-Stompin' Music"
Bohannon

"Shotgun Shuffle"
KC & the Sunshine Band

"(If You Want It)
Do It Yourself"
Gloria Gaynor

"Dreaming a Dream"
Crown Heights Affair

"Ease on down the Road"
Consumer Rapport

BUMP BUS STOP

"It Only Takes a Minute"
Tavares

"Do It Anyway You Wanna"
People's Choice

"Peace Pipe"
B.T. Express

"Fight the Power"
The Isley Brothers

"7-6-5-4-3-2-1
(Blow Your Whistle)"
Gary Toms Empire

REGGAE

"Funky Kingston"
Toots and the Maytals

"The Harder They Come"
Jimmy Cliff

"Israelites"
Desmond Dekker & the Aces

"Trenchtown Rock"
Bob Marley & the Wailers

"The World Turned Upside Down"
Joe Higgs

DISCO ALL STARS

"Can't Get Enough of Your Love, Babe"
Barry White

"Rock Your Baby"
George McRae

"Shining Star"
Earth, Wind & Fire

"Love Rollercoaster"
Ohio Players

"Fight the Power"
Isley Brothers

PHILLY SOUND

"Backstabbers"
O'Jays

"T.S.O.P."
MFSB

"Bad Luck"
Harold Melvin & the Blue Notes

"I Can't Stop Dancing"
Archie Bell & the Drells

"I Love Music"
O'Jays

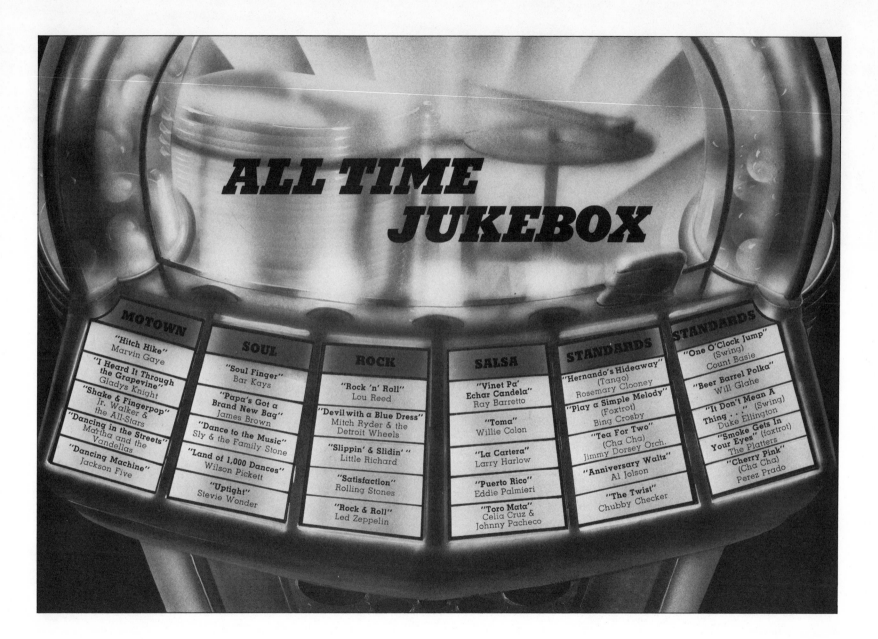

ALL TIME JUKEBOX

MOTOWN

"Hitch Hike"
Marvin Gaye

"I Heard It Through
the Grapevine"
Gladys Knight

"Shake & Fingerpop"
Jr. Walker &
the All-Stars

"Dancing in the Streets"
Martha and the
Vandellas

"Dancing Machine"
Jackson Five

SOUL

"Soul Finger"
Bar Kays

"Papa's Got a
Brand New Bag"
James Brown

"Dance to the Music"
Sly & the Family Stone

"Land of 1,000 Dances"
Wilson Pickett

"Uptight"
Stevie Wonder

ROCK

"Rock 'n' Roll"
Lou Reed

"Devil with a Blue Dress"
Mitch Ryder & the
Detroit Wheels

"Slippin' & Slidin'"
Little Richard

"Satisfaction"
Rolling Stones

"Rock & Roll"
Led Zeppelin

SALSA

"Vinet Pa'
Echar Candela"
Ray Barretto

"Toma"
Willie Colon

"La Cartera"
Larry Harlow

"Puerto Rico"
Eddie Palmieri

"Toro Mata"
Celia Cruz &
Johnny Pacheco

STANDARDS

"Hernando's Hideaway"
(Tango)
Rosemary Clooney

"Play a Simple Melody"
(Foxtrot)
Bing Crosby

"Tea For Two"
(Cha Cha)
Jimmy Dorsey Orch.

"Anniversary Waltz"
Al Jolson

"The Twist"
Chubby Checker

STANDARDS

"One O'Clock Jump"
(Swing)
Count Basie

"Beer Barrel Polka"
Will Glahe

"It Don't Mean A
Thing . . ." (Swing)
Duke Ellington

"Smoke Gets In
Your Eyes" (foxtrot)
The Platters

"Cherry Pink"
(Cha Cha)
Perez Prado

CREDITS

Editorial researcher and production manager: Linda Ross

Picture researcher: Karen Mullarky; assistance by Carol Raskin-Ward

Copy editor: Barbara Downey

Proofreaders: Catharine Norton, Madeline Pober

Production: Karen Becker, Ren Deaton, Paul Miller, Adele Prosdócimi, Nancy Rinehart, Maria Wang

Technical advisers: Teddy Lee, Derék Lewis, Karen Lustgarten

Cover illustration: Mick Haggerty

"No Sober Person Dances": photos by Waring Abbott

"The Method behind the Madness": photos p 16, by Antonin Kratochvil; photo p 18, 19, 20 by Waring Abbott

"Disco Tech": photo p 26 by Max Hellweg

"Confessions of the Disco Kid": photos p 30, 32=33 by Max Hellweg

The New York Hustle: photos by Waring Abbott

Hustle and Bump Flips: figures p 37-79 by Robert Grossman

Hustle Charts: charts p 38-39 compiled by Karen Lustgarten and Ralph Lew, design by Paul Miller

"Disco Stars": photos of the Isley Brothers (p 47), the Ritchie Family (p 53) and Disco-Tex (p 67) by Waring Abbott; the Lockers (p 59) by David Alexander; the Kay Gees (p 64) by Max Hellweg, Tito Puente (p 71) by Wendi Lombardi

The Bump: photo p 60 by Neal Preston; photos p 62—left by Michael Zagaris, right by Charles Gatewood, Magnum Photos; photos p 63 by Waring Abbott

"Disco 'Round the World": thanks to Joe Cunningham (Japan), Jay Grossman (Mexico), Paul Gambaccini and friend (France), and to *Billboard* and *Melody Maker* magazines

Reggae: photos p 86, 88-91 by Michael Dobo. Special thanks to Toots Hibbert and Island Records

Salsa: photos p 92, 94-97 by David Haas. Special thanks to Willie Colon, Iris Feliciano, La Conspiracion and Marty Arret of the Corso

Soul: photos p 98, 100-103 by Neal Preston. Special thanks to Damita Jo Freeman

The L. A. Hustle: photos p 104, 106-109 by Lawrence Bartone. Special thanks to Karen Lustgarten

"Slipped Disco": illustration p 110 by Greg Scott. Special thanks to Dr. Gilbert Kucera

"It Seems We've Stood and Danced like This Before": photos p 114, 117-118, 122 from the Bettmann Archive, Inc.; p 121 by Cornell Capa, Magnum Photos; p 124 by Paul Schutzer, Time-Life Picture Agency; p 125 by Jim Marshall; p 126 by Charles Harbutt, Magnum Photos. Research sources: *The Unembarrassed Muse: The Popular Arts in America*, by Russell Nye, Dial Press, N. Y. 1971; *Guinness Book of World Records*, edited by Norris and Ross McWhirter, Sterling Publishing Co., N. Y. 1973; *How to Dance*, by Thomas E. Parson, Barnes & Noble Books, N. Y. 1969; *This Is Ballroom Dance*, by Lois Ellfeldt and Virgil L. Morton, National Press Books, Palo Alto 1974; *The Oxford History of the American People*, Volume Three, by Samuel Eliot Morison, New American Library, N. Y. 1972; *Social Dance: A Short History*, by A. H. Franks, Routledge and Kegan Paul, London 1963; "A History of Recreational Social Dance in the United States," by John Green Youman, a thesis presented to the faculty of the Graduate School, University of Southern California, 1966. Special thanks to Carl Gottlieb

"The Wedding/Prom/Bar Mitzvah Survival Guide": photos p 128, 130, 134, 138 by Max Hellweg. Research verification through technical advisers and dance texts as above. Special thanks to Teddy and Ingrid Lee. Dance diagrams prepared by Linda Ross

"The Keep on Dancin' All Time Jukebox": jukebox by Phil Carroll. Special thanks to Michael Ochs, Ed Ward; Ruel Mills of Kingston Productions, San Francisco; John Jensen of KMPX, San Francisco

Parts of this book first appeared in the Dancing Madness supplement, Issue 194, *Rolling Stone* magazine.